Ketogenic diet and exercise plan

Burn fat, gain muscle, have more energy

With simple keto meal prep

By: Susan Katz

TABLE OF CONTENTS

Introduction

Burn 15 pounds in 20 minutes every day! No work needed! Try this weird trick that tricks your body into burning fat!

How many of us have seen some version of the above ad while browsing the internet? How many of us have been unfortunate enough to actually believe its claims and ended up clicking on it? Losing weight and being physically fit is one of the top wishes everybody has no matter where they're from. Like everything else, choosing the correct way to go about things is daunting just because there's so much information out there. There's a ton of evidence to support something and just as much, seemingly, which refute it. Then there is the litany of terms one needs to become familiar with when adopting any new diet plan or information.

Paleo, Keto, LCHF, HCLF, Atkins, Weight Watchers, South Beach, No carbs after 6 PM, carbs only after 6 PM, cardio vs strength training, training on an empty stomach, protein, carbs, fat.....and on and on it goes. Even if you do become comfortable with all these terms, losing weight isn't guaranteed. You might see some results but making sure the results remain is another matter entirely.

Funnily enough, it is the very existence of so many diet plans and training programs that spawn newer, shinier diets. People are always searching for a better, more "guaranteed" plan and naturally, the market rises to fill their needs. These days, given the number of content channels out there, its easy to be bombarded with media on pretty much any topic of your choice, no matter how bizarre. Even as we speak, there are probably videos being uploaded out there detailing how you can lose weight using telekinesis or some such.

Vegans and vegetarians face further issues since a lot of diets readily assume their audience has no problem consuming meat and dairy. Generally speaking, following a diet plan while living a vegan lifestyle is difficult enough and all this additional confusion is the last thing you need. How did food become so complicated? More importantly, how does one unravel it?

Back to Basics

The answer is simple: Ignore the noise and head back to the basics. Our bodies are far more resilient than we give them credit for and there is no need to treat them like porcelain dolls (assuming you don't have a debilitating disease of course). You don't need an extremely fancy diet which causes you to worry about what to and what not to eat constantly. You just need to learn some basics about how the body burns food as fuel and how by understanding this process and following some simple principles, you can make any diet work.

The Ketogenic diet is one of those basic diet plans, believe it or not. The name for this diet might be newfangled but the principles of this diet have existed in some form or another for a long time. Why? Because it's common sense! There's nothing fancy about it unless you wish to make it so.

This book is going to give you the lowdown on the Ketogenic (Keto for short) diet. We will be by looking at the basics of using food as fuel and examine the science behind the diet's effectiveness. For all you vegans out there, the advice given in this book, especially regarding nutrition and exercise, applies fully to you as well. The only additional item you need to take care of is figuring out are vegan sources of protein and fat. While fat is easily sourced via seeds and oils, protein is tougher. You need not worry though since a list of vegan protein sources along with supplements are provided.

Along the way, we will also look at specific situations and exercise plans you can implement straight away, no matter which fitness level you're at. There will need to be some level of complexity depending on your goals (for example an athlete versus a rank beginner) but this book will walk you through all of it, step by step.

We will also be busting some myths along the way and vegans need not worry, we'll be covering how the Keto diet can fit seamlessly into your lifestyle!

So sit back and enjoy!

Chapter 1: The Basics of Nutrition

Before we dive into the Keto diet, it is essential that you understand some basics about how our bodies burn the food we consume to provide us with energy and why some foods are good for us and some bad. Understanding this information will help you see why the Keto diet works, far more easily. In addition, you will also be able to evaluate the merits and drawbacks of any other diet you might encounter.

In this chapter, we will break down how the composition of the food you eat affects your health and why your mother was right when she told you to finish your veggies when you were a kid. If you've ever been confused about protein, carbohydrates, vitamins, minerals etc and how they function to aid your well-being, this chapter will have all the answers for you!

Nutrition and Nutrients

So what is nutrition? After all, no matter which diet we choose, good nutrition is what we're after. While all of us have some idea of what it is, it's better to define it.

The World Health Organization defines nutrition as follows: Nutrition is the intake of food, considered in relation to the body's dietary needs. Good nutrition – an adequate, well-balanced diet combined with regular physical activity – is a cornerstone of good health. Poor nutrition can lead to reduced immunity, increased susceptibility to disease, impaired physical and mental development, and reduced productivity.[1] ("Nutrition", 2019).

Now that that's out of the way, we can surmise that nutrition is essentially how we feed ourselves. We can do this in a good or a bad way.

Balanced Diets

A balanced diet, from the definition above, simply refers to eating foods from different food groups as part of our daily food intake. The different food groups, roughly speaking, are:

1. Vegetables
2. Meats
3. Grains

[1] Nutrition. 2019. Retrieved from https://www.who.int/topics/nutrition/en/

4. Fruits

5. Dairy

Of course, lifestyle choices do affect our ability to follow this advice. This is where it's important to remember how resilient our bodies are. If you're vegan and choose to forego items 2 and 5, this doesn't mean you're condemning yourself to malnutrition. While your nutrition might not be at its most optimum state, this is hardly something to fuss over.

What is far more important to understand is that a balanced diet is recommended because each food group is abundant in a different type of nutrient. Nutrients are what make up all the food we consume. Thus, whether you eat different food groups in a balanced manner or not, what you should be doing is getting a good mix of nutrients in your diet.

Nutrients

There are six major forms of nutrients. They can be listed as:

- Carbohydrates: Also called Carbs
- Proteins
- Fats
- Vitamins
- Mineral

- Water

Before everything else, we need to acknowledge that the most important nutrient is water. Our bodies are 60% water and our brains are composed of 70% water. Simply put, without clean, drinkable water, we simply will not survive. No matter which diet you decide to adopt, drinking adequate water is essential. The Mayo Clinic recommends 3.7 liters of water per day for adult men and 2.7 liters per day for adult women[2] ("Water: How much should you drink every day?" 2019).

Each of the above nutrients has a certain caloric profile, that is, they provide different amounts of energy to our bodies when burned. Proteins, carbs and fats provide the large majority of energy when burned. Vitamins and minerals are responsible for other functions while providing trace amounts of energy. They are responsible for a number of things such as bone health, immune system health and repairing cellular damage.

When it comes to understanding weight loss and evaluating the merits of a new diet, our main focus rests on proteins, fats and carbs. Let us now take a closer look at each of these nutrients.

---

[2] Water: How much should you drink everyday?. (2019). Retrieved from https://www.mayoclinic.org/healthy-lifestyle/nutrition-and-healthy-eating/in-depth/water/art-20044256

Protein

Proteins are the building blocks of our bodies. They are what help build muscle and tissue. Our bodies convert external proteins into internal ones, like enzymes, and this is how our muscles are maintained and built.

Proteins themselves are made of amino acids, of which there are multiple types. Without going into great detail, animal protein contains a denser distribution of amino acids than plant protein. In other words, if you eat meat, you're likelier to receive your entire amino acid intake in fewer meals as opposed to eating only plants or plant-based food.

Vegans need to eat a wider variety of food to achieve their protein needs. No matter which diet you choose to follow, it is essential you meet your daily protein requirement. Given their function in maintaining muscle, this point should be self-explanatory. The amount of proteins you need to consume daily depends on your lifestyle goals and this will be explored later in this book.

Carbohydrates

Carbs are one of our primary sources of energy. While they do have other essential functions, their main purpose is to provide us with energy to go about our day. Chemically speaking, carbs are simple sugars and starches, which when broken down, turn into glucose which feeds our energy needs.

If you've been paying even a little attention to food-related literature, you will be aware of how bad sugars are supposed to be for you. Now, it is important to realize that naturally occurring sugars, such as those in carbs, are not bad for you. In fact, sugar in appropriate quantities is a part of a balanced diet and you should not be striving to avoid "all" sugar.

If this is confusing, don't worry, we'll cover all this in a later chapter. For now, it is important for you to understand that carbs contain sugar and in this form, sugar is not bad for you but is actually essential for healthy body functions.

Fat

The technically correct scientific term for fat is "lipids" but for simplicity's sake, we will be referring to them as fat or fats. Again, thanks to the influence of popular literature, it is important to note right at the outset: Fat does not make you fat. Neither is fat the only thing that causes you to put on weight. This is an especially relevant point if you are to follow the Keto diet.

Fats also have the same function as carbs in that they are a fuel source, primarily. Fats come in two varieties, saturated and unsaturated. Unsaturated fats, such as coconut and olive oil, are good for you in the right quantities but saturated fats are a bit more controversial.

Thus far, nutritionists agree that saturated fat in excess quantities is harmful but some level of saturated fats are necessary for a balanced diet. Consumed in excess, saturated fats cause hardening of the arteries, that is when arteries get blocked with fat, and cause heart disease. The advice to avoid red meat originates from this fact. Red meat has high amounts of saturated fat and excess consumption will lead to all sorts of unsavory diseases. However, avoiding it entirely isn't appropriate either.

This principle is true of pretty much all kinds of food (with one notable exception) and this is why a lot of confusion crops up. Most people think of nutrition in an either/or sort of way and unfortunately, our bodies have not evolved with an either/or logic. The truth is, everything needs to consumed in the appropriate quantity. As long as you stick to the appropriate levels, things are good for you. Cross these limits and its bad. When it comes to nutrition, too much of a good thing is a very real consequence. It is important you approach any diet plan with this philosophy.

Many diets demonize a particular nutrient or macronutrient and this is simply lacking in scientific fact. So the next time you see a blanket statement that says "All fats are bad" or "all carbs are unhealthy," know that they are false.

Energy

We've seen in the previous section how our bodies have three primary sources of energy: Proteins, Carbs and Fat. Proteins are probably the most important of the lot because of their role in maintaining our muscles via amino acids. Carbs and fat form the remainder of our fuel sources.

The next bit to understand is that the energy profile of these three is not equal. In other words, one unit of protein does not generate the same amount of energy as one unit of carbs or 1 unit of fat. The energy released by these nutrients are measured in kilocalories (kcal). While technically not the same, in common reference, a kilocalorie is called a "Calorie". Moving forward, to keep things simple, we will refer to this in the same way. Just remember that when we say Calorie, we're talking about kilocalories for simplicity's sake and to avoid confusion with other sources.

The caloric profile of the three major nutrients is listed in the table below:

Nutrient	Calories per gram
Proteins	4
Carbohydrates	4
Fats	9

As you can see, fats are more calorie dense than the other two. In other words, to gain the same amount of Calories, you need to eat less fat than carbs or proteins. This is an important building block of the Keto diet.

As we go about our day and consume food, our body keeps burning it and realizing energy, via Calories, as per the table above. If we eat as much food, or Calories, as our body needs during the day, we feel sated and can function at a normal level. If we consume less, we will feel a bit hungry but this isn't a disaster. There is a healthy limit up to which we can consume less than our required Caloric amount per day. Drop below this limit and your body starts breaking down and when prolonged, this becomes unhealthy and leads to all sorts of unwanted consequences.

Similarly there is a healthy limit above your Caloric needs up to which you can consume excess Calories. Go above this limit and you'll, once again, be damaging yourself. Simply put, eat below the healthy limit and you suffer from malnutrition. Eat above the limit and you suffer from obesity. If there was a way to summarize the process of maintaining a healthy weight, that would be it.

Weight Loss and Fat Loss

Most people, when they pick up a book like this, have the aim of weight loss in their mind. What they should be concerned about instead is fat loss. The best way to think of this is as follows: While all fat loss is weight loss, not all weight loss is fat loss.

To examine why this is the case, we need to look at what happens when we eat too much or too little. Let's tackle the former first.

When you consume an excess of calories, your body after burning off whatever it needs to function for the day, has to decide what to do with the surplus calories. What it usually does is, it stores these excess calories as glycogen. This is to ensure you have a decent reserve of energy in case an emergency arises. Glycogen storage is accompanied by a proportional amount of water storage, usually in a 1:3 ratio.

Once the Glycogen stores are filled, if there are any remaining calories left they get stored as fat. This is the fat which shows up in various parts of our body and when it becomes excessive, causes us to reach for a book like this. This is how eating too much makes you fat. Note that at no point does your body differentiate between a Calorie coming from carbs versus protein versus fat. A Calorie is a Calorie no matter where it comes from.

The above narrative oversimplifies the process but as an introduction, this is all you need to know, unless you wish to become a nutritionist. Let us now look at what happens when you run a deficit, that is, you eat less than what you need.

When this happens, your body has a very simple plan. It burns off its stores with priority given to glycogen first and then fat, failing which it will turn to muscle to meet its energy needs. The reason behind this order is not relevant, again, unless you wish to specialize in nutritional science. Suffice to say that, this mechanism is what has evolved in us and serves us well. The body, in this manner always has backup energy to keep you fueled for a certain period, until you refuel.

Given this prioritization of what to burn first, it becomes an easy task for us to determine the best way to lose fat (since we do not wish to lose muscle). We maintain a caloric deficit (that is, eat less than what we need) and once the glycogen stores are depleted, our fat burns off. Of course, we need to take care to not eat too less or else our muscle gets burned as well in the process.

You see, this is the difference between referring to weight loss versus fat loss. Weight loss includes a number of things. If you drink less water, your weight decreases. You could be at your ideal, healthy "weight" and still be unhealthy. The key thing to remember is that you need to minimize the amount of fat in your body and maximize lean muscle. This is where your exercise and diet play a vital role. If your goal is mere weight loss, then starve yourself for a few days. This is the easiest way to lose"weight". However, think of how much damage you're doing to yourself in the process. This is also why starving yourself, in the long term, is never the answer if you're overweight. Controlled caloric deficits are the way to go.

Exercise

It is entirely possible to lose fat without exercise. Around 80% of your fat loss is dependent on your diet. Why then, you might wonder, should you exercise? After all, isn’t the gym one of the most strenuous places to visit? Most people would love the extra hour or so of sleep they would gain.

Exercise has innumerable benefits for your body and all of these are very well known. From a nutrition perspective though, exercise plays a very important role. It helps build muscle. You see, the greater the amount of muscle you have, the easier it is to burn fat and tougher it is to put fat on. Let's see how this works.

When you eat something your body has the option of choosing how it wishes to use this energy. It could use this energy to fuel you (thereby burning all of it) or it could choose to set it aside as either glycogen or fat. The more muscle you have, the more the food that you consume is redirected to feed those muscles and thus less is left over for storage. Why? Well, given that your strength and conditioning is pretty high, the body reasons you don't need as much as emergency storage.

Think of it this way: In a workplace, the more capable someone is at their job, the less likely it is that you, as a manager, need to worry about providing backup to that person should they fail their task. If your team happens to have someone who isn't pulling their weight though, you need to set aside more resources to help compensate for that lag. Your body reasons much the same way.

This doesn't mean the answer is to simply pack on more muscle until you burst. It's just that you need to consistently exercise and make sure your physical and cardiovascular systems are in a healthy state. Once you do this and eat right, the muscle building takes care of itself and in turn any food you eat builds more muscle and your fat content reduces.

Thus, you see, your body helps you stay lean the more you exercise. If you choose to not exercise, your body doesn't see the need to divert more energy towards helping your muscles since they don't require as much energy and neither are they greater in number. Thus the weight you will lose by eating less and not exercising will be an equal proportion of fat and muscle. The net result is you'll lose weight but strength as well. Aesthetically, you'll look about the same, just weaker. Exercise is extremely important to avoid this state of affairs.

Diet

While it's all fine to say that you need to eat less than you burn to lose weight, what you eat plays an important role. There is a very real difference between good Calories and bad Calories.

Calories from junk food is a prime example of bad Calories. While, in the short run, you will lose weight by eating less junk food than you need to burn, you will be putting a huge amount of stress on your internal systems thanks to the highly processed, chemically altered nature of these foods. Think of it this way: You can be the healthiest looking person alive but still have organ failure. While this is exaggerating it by a lot, it highlights an important point regarding health: You need to be healthy both inside and the outside.

When choosing a diet, you need to begin with proteins as this is absolutely needed for a healthy lifestyle. Consuming protein will help you build and maintain muscle and the amount you ingest, as mentioned previously, will depend on what your goals are. We'll list the exact numbers later but for now, suffice to say, an athlete will need far more protein than someone who exercises twice a week and has a sedentary job.

Once you've determined this, you then have a choice of either balancing carbs and fat or prioritizing one over the other. All choices have their pros and cons and it is here, finally, we arrive at the point of the Ketogenic diet.

The Keto diet prioritizes fats over carbs for a number of reasons we'll be looking at in the next chapter. Before going there though, you still need to keep in mind that if you overeat on the Keto diet, you will still gain weight. The diet is not a magic bullet and the principle guiding fat loss, that is maintaining a caloric deficit, still applies. You will need to exercise when following this diet as well, needless to say.

So, now that we understand the basic principles, let's dive in and look at the Ketogenic diet and why this is the most effective diet for fat loss.

Chapter 2: The Ketogenic Diet

The Ketogenic diet is, contrary to popular perception, one of the oldest diets out there. Originally developed in the 1920s as a treatment for children suffering from epilepsy [1] (Mandal, 2019), the Ketogenic diet eventually went mainstream thanks to the effects people started noticing in body composition, apart from the impact on epilepsy itself.

In this chapter we're going to take a deep look at the science behind all of it and why the diet works as spectacularly as it does. We will also see the different modifications you can make to it to suit your lifestyle.

Principles

The Ketogenic diet emphasizes the importance of fats in the

---

[1] Mandal, A. (2019). History of the Ketogenic Diet. Retrieved from https://www.news-medical.net/health/History-of-the-Ketogenic-Diet.aspx

diet over carbs given a predetermined level of protein. This diet is shown to offer a number of health benefits, from reducing obesity and epilepsy to even minimizing the chances of contracting cancer and managing diabetes or Alzheimer's disease.

These claims are not simply conjured out of thin air. Keto has been around as long as it has so it's is one of the most intensely studied and dissected diet out there. These studies are largely responsible for dispensing with the notion that eating fat makes us fat. Let us look at some of the more popular studies to better examine the health effects of Keto.

Obesity

A study conducted in 2003 compared the effects of a low carb diet (Keto) versus a low-fat diet on obesity (Foster et al., 2003). Sixty-three subjects were randomly placed into two groups: one which followed a low-fat diet and another which followed a low carb diet.

The results are summarized below:[2] (Foster et al., 2003)

In the analysis in which baseline values were carried

---

[2] Foster, G., Wyatt H., Hill, J., McGuckin, B., Brill, C., & Mohammed, B. et al. (2003). A Randomized Trial of a Low-Carbohydrate Diet for Obesity. New England Journal Of Medicine, 348(21), 2082-2090. doi: 10.1056/nejmoa022207[29]

forward in the case of missing values, the group on the low-carbohydrate diet had lost significantly more weight than the group on the conventional diet at 3 months (P=0.001) and 6 months (P=0.02), but the difference in weight loss was not statistically significant at 12 months.

In other words at the 6-month mark, the results clearly showed the subjects on the low carb diet had lost more weight than the other group. However, attrition is high, the study was inconclusive over a period of 12 months. Additionally, the low carb group had greater improvement in triglycerides and HDL.

The efficacy of a low carb diet was studied on healthy women as well to prove that such a diet isn't meant only for those suffering from physical ailments.[3] (Brehm, Seeley, Daniels & D'Alessio, 2003). This study tracked 53 healthy but moderately obese women over a period of 6 months. Subjects were randomized into either a low carb diet group or a low-fat diet group.

The results were just as conclusive and statistically

---

[3] Brehm, B., Seeley, R., Daniels, S., & D'Alessio, D. (2003). A Randomized Trial Comparing a Very Low Carbohydrate Diet and a Calorie-Restricted Low Fat Diet on Body Weight and Cardiovascular Risk Factors in Healthy Women. *The Journal Of Clinical Endocrinalogy & Metabolism*, 88(4), 1617-1623. doi: 10.1210/jc2002-021480

significant as the previous study. The subjects in the low carb group lost, on average, 19 lbs while the women in the other group lost, on average, 8.6 lbs overall. Also, once again, the triglycerides and HDL levels were found to be better in the low carb group. In conclusion, the authors had this to say:

Based on these data, a very low carbohydrate diet is more effective than a low-fat diet for short-term weight loss and, over 6 months, is not associated with deleterious effects on important cardiovascular risk factors in healthy women

Diabetes

A study in 2006 aimed to observe the effects of low carb, restricted diet on patients suffering from Type 2 diabetes. 102 patients were randomized into two groups, again, one following a low fat and the other following a low carb diet plan for a period of 6 months[4] (Daly et al., 2006).

The results of this study speak for themselves: (Daly et al., 2006)

Weight loss was greater in the low-carbohydrate (LC) group (−3.55 ± 0.63, mean ± sem) vs. −0.92 ± 0.40 kg, P =

---

[4] Daly, M., Paisey, R., Paisey, R., Millward, B., Eccles, C., & Williams, K. et al. (2006). Short-term effects of severe dietary carbohydrate-restriction advice in Type 2 diabetes-a randomized controlled trial. *Diabetic Medicine,* 23(1), 15-20. doi: 10.1111/j.1464-5491.2005.01760.x

0.001) and cholesterol : high-density lipoprotein (HDL) ratio improved (−0.48 ± 0.11 vs. −0.10 ± 0.10, P = 0.01). However, relative saturated fat intake was greater (13.9 ± 0.71 vs. 11.0 ± 0.47% of dietary intake, P < 0.001), although absolute intakes were moderate.

Alzheimer's

A 2006 study found significant evidence that the ketogenic diet does have effects on our brain's neural structure and that this may help reduce the debilitating effect of diseases where cellular level changes affect healthy functioning adversely[5] (Gasior et al., 2006).

The conclusions of this study were significant: (Gasior et al., 2006)

It has long been recognized that the ketogenic diet is associated with increased circulating levels of ketone bodies, which represent a more efficient fuel in the brain, and there may also be increased numbers of brain mitochondria. It is plausible that the enhanced energy production capacity resulting from these effects would confer neurons with greater ability to resist metabolic challenges……

---

[5] Gasior, M., Rogawski, M.A., & Hartman, A. L. (2006). Neuroprotective and disease-modifying effects of the ketogenic diet. *Behavioural Pharmacology*, 17(5-6), 431-9.

Although each of the aforementioned alternatives is still early in development, the idea of developing the ketogenic diet in a 'pill' is very attractive and may be approachable.

Brain Cancer

A 2007 study indicated the effectiveness of the Keto diet as an alternative option for malignant brain cancer. While, obviously, not a cure for the disease, the reduction in tumor growth was statistically significant [6](Zhou et al., 2007).

Below are the results observed in the study:11[7](Zhou et al., 2007)

KetoCal administered in restricted amounts significantly decreased the intracerebral growth of the CT-2A and U87-MG tumors by about 65% and 35%, respectively, and significantly enhanced health and survival relative to that of the control groups receiving the standard low fat/high

---

[6] Zhou, W., Mukherjee, P., Kiebish, M. A., Markis, W. T., Mantis, J. G., & Seyfried, T. N. (2007). The calorically restricted ketogenic diet, effective alternative therapy for malignant brain cancer. *Nutrition & Metabolism*, 4, 5. doi:10.1186/1743-7075-4-5

[7] Zhou, W., Mukherjee, P., Kiebish, M. A., Markis, W. T., Mantis, J. G., & Seyfried, T. N. (2007). The calorically restricted ketogenic diet, effective alternative therapy for malignant brain cancer. *Nutrition & Metabolism*, 4, 5. doi:10.1186/1743-7075-4-5

carbohydrate diet. The restricted KetoCal diet reduced plasma glucose levels while elevating plasma ketone body (beta-hydroxybutyrate) levels. Tumor microvessel density was less in the calorically restricted KetoCal groups than in the calorically unrestricted control groups. Moreover, gene expression for the mitochondrial enzymes, beta-hydroxybutyrate dehydrogenase and succinyl-CoA: 3-ketoacid CoA transferase, was lower in the tumors than in the contralateral normal brain suggesting that these brain tumors have reduced ability to metabolize ketone bodies for energy.

The conclusion of this study was that due to the tumor's growth being dependent on glucose, a caloric restriction combined with a high-fat diet slowed the growth of the tumors and that the diet could function as an alternative therapy [8] (Zhou et al., 2007)

Acne

Yes, even common acne was found to be minimized greatly when following the ketogenic diet. While this study wasn't as

---

[8] Zhou, W., Mukherjee, P., Kiebish, M. A., Markis, W. T., Mantis, J. G., & Seyfried, T. N. (2007). The calorically restricted ketogenic diet, an effective alternative therapy for malignant brain cancer. *Nutrition & Metabolism*, 4, 5. doi:10.1186/1743-7075-4-5

conclusive as possible, the results were definitely significant[9] (Paoli et al., 2012).

As must be obvious by now, the keto diet is highly effective in not just losing weight but also in mitigating the debilitating effects of many diseases. The journal articles cited here are just the tip of the iceberg when it comes to the number of studies performed on the diet.

We've already seen how the ketogenic diet is a low carb, high-fat diet. Let's now take a closer look at how it works physically and why it is as effective as it is.

Ketosis

This section could have also been named "the secret of Ketogenic diets". Ketosis is why you will lose weight when following this diet. What is Ketosis though and how is it induced? Why is it induced only on a high-fat diet? How does it work? We'll examine the answers in the following sections.

[9] Paoli, A., Grimaldi, K., Toniolo, L., Canato, M., Bianco, A., & Fratter, A. (2012). Nutrition and Acne: Therapeutic Potential of Ketogenic Diets. *Skin Pharmacology And Physiology*, 25(3), 111-117. doi: 10.1159/000336404

What is it?

Ketosis is a normal bodily function wherein the body starts burning fat instead of glucose in order to produce energy. As we saw earlier, glucose is the body's primary fuel source and the first in the order of priority when it comes to burning in order to produce energy.

When there is a lack of glucose, the body needs an alternate fuel source and fat provides it. As fat is burned, there is a rise of acids called Ketones and their presence in the bloodstream is an indication that the body is burning fat instead of glucose. Ketones are excreted via urine and are a natural by-product of ketosis.

Safety

Ketosis, if induced, is a fully normal bodily process and you have nothing to fear from it. Excessive levels of it, however, point to issues with the body's ability to produce and use insulin and is an indicator of diabetes.

Indeed, in patients suffering from type 1 diabetes, extreme ketosis is more likely to develop. Ketosis can be safely induced by following a low carb diet. Carbs are a primary source of glucose, given that they are sugars as we saw previously, and once you restrict them, the body is forced to burn fat instead.

Again, this does not mean you starve yourself. Fasting for a day is fine and is an ancient method to induce ketosis in the body but prolonging this state of affairs in unhealthy. This is why it is essential you substitute the Calories lost due to the carb restriction with calories from fats while maintaining an appropriate protein level in your diet.

Ketosis and Ketoacidosis

Ketosis should not be confused with Ketoacidosis which is an extreme condition of ketosis. As ketone levels go beyond safe parameters in the bloodstream, the blood becomes highly acidified and this is a serious medical condition which requires emergency intervention.

This phenomenon is usually observed in people suffering from Type 1 diabetes. While there are instances of it occurring in people with Type 2 diabetes, it is very rare. Now, if you suffer from diabetes, you might be wondering if the Ketogenic diet is safe for you?

Effect on Diabetes

As we saw from the medical studies in the previous section, the keto diet is perfectly safe for patients with Type 2 diabetes. People suffering from Type 1 diabetes will need to consult their doctor on the best course of action to take.

Due to the diabetic condition, where the body does not process insulin effectively, being as it is, doctors often prescribe a low carb diet for patients in order to prevent blood sugar levels from spiking. Having said that, Type 2 diabetes patients need to constantly monitor the ketone level within their bloodstream due to the danger of ketoacidosis.

Ketones do show up in the urine but the best way to measure their level is via a blood test. There are a number of self-testing kits available which do the job excellently. Healthy and desired levels of ketones in the blood amount to 0.5-3 mmol/L. If you wish to measure them via your urine then indicator strips will do the job.

Any person following the keto diet can choose to track their ketone levels to determine whether they are in ketosis or not. There are some other symptoms as well as we shall see next.

Other Symptoms of Ketosis

- Bad breath: Higher levels of ketones mean greater levels of acetone which gives your breath a distinctly fruity flavor. You might need to brush multiple times a day or use sugar-free gum to combat this.

- Fast Weight Loss: After initially adopting the keto diet, depending on how much weight you need to lose, you will see a drastic drop in your weight. This is not fat reduction but simply water weight being shed. Remember, in the previous chapter, we saw how water needs to be stored as glucose levels increase? Well, if glucose levels decrease there's no need for excess water so your body gets rid of it.

- Decreased energy initially: If you've never had a low carb diet before, adjusting to it takes time. During this time, your body, which is used to burning high amounts of glucose to fuel you, is still looking for glucose simply because it is used to it. Once it figures out there's no glucose it starts to burn fat instead and this is when your energy levels rise. Most dieters report this "keto fog" lasting a week at most. Switching diets over the weekend is a good idea in order to combat this.

- Less hunger pangs: On the keto diet, you will see that your hunger isn't as ferocious as it usually is. While the exact reason for this is not known, many dieters have reported this event for it to be statistically significant. Dieticians think this might be the ketones changing the way our brains process hunger.

- Changing bowel movements: Constipation and diarrhea are side effects when beginning the keto diet. Due to the reduced number of carbs, and the fiber they provide, your bowel movements usually suffer. This can be mitigated by eating lots of leafy greens or taking a fiber supplement. Getting the amount right takes some trial and error and it is in this period when you might suffer from diarrhea due to taking too much fiber.

So as you can see there are a number of ways to tell if you're in ketosis or not. Getting into ketosis is what the keto diet is all about and it pays to track your state when adopting the diet for the first time.

Ketogenic Foods

So now that we've looked at the science behind the keto diet, understood ketosis and its importance and are up to speed with the basics of nutrition, it's time to finally dig into what to eat when following the ketogenic diet. This section will list everything you should eat and what you should avoid. Vegans will also find plenty of options here so if you are one, you need not worry!

Right off the bat, you need to understand that all chemically-processed foods should be avoided like the plague. This is not a ketogenic diet rule as much as a common sense rule. Highly processed foods contain chemicals which cause harm and you need to avoid these foods. Examples include TV dinners, frozen pizza, fast food, sugary soft drinks and other chemically processed food. A good rule of thumb is to have whole foods as much as possible. For example, cheese is a processed food but a lot of cheese isn't chemically or artificially processed.

Foods labeled "diet" or "low fat" should be avoided as well since more often than not they are chemically altered. Any meat that has had hormones injected into it, needless to say, does not fit the bill. Eating organic as much as possible is the best way forward. This isn't always practical so at the very least, avoid the overly sugary and obviously chemically processed foods for now.

Let's now look at what you should eat on the ketogenic diet.

Meat

Meat lovers rejoice! All kinds of meat, red, white, steak, chicken and turkey is perfectly compatible with the keto diet. Protein plays an important role in the diet. While the primary aim is to reduce your overall fat levels, a secondary aim is to increase lean body mass or muscle. This in turn helps the primary objective.

Meat is an excellent source of protein. Take care to see that the meat you purchase is of good quality and is hormone-free as much as possible. Also, opt for leaner cuts. Despite the keto diet being a high-fat diet, it isn't a free license for you to load up on fatty cuts. The fats found in meat are usually saturated fats and an excess of this is not healthy.

Opting for chicken breasts instead of thighs, for example, is making a good choice.

Fatty Fish

Fish make the cut as well on the keto diet. Salmon, tuna and mackerel are examples of excellent, healthy fish you can consume. A cheaper option would be sardines which can be purchased canned or fresh.

When eating fish higher on the food chain like salmon or tuna, you must be careful to avoid mercury poisoning which may occur due to over-consumption. A similar warning applies to smoked salmon. While delicious, the smoking process does cause some chemicals to form which are toxic in large quantities.

Eggs

Eggs are your go-to protein source. Make sure you eat the yolk as well since the majority of the protein is found there. While the yolk does increase your harmful cholesterol, with regular exercise and a diet which is healthy overall, the harmful effects are greatly reduced to the point of not existing.

Ideally, you should consume omega-3, organic free range eggs but again if this is not an option, try to consume eggs which are as close to organic as possible.

Butter and Cream

Off all the foods on the keto diet, these are the ones people have the most trouble consuming. Years of conditioning about how fat is bad for you and how it clogs your arteries have lead people to swearing off these completely healthy options.

Moderation is key here and again, choosing the best sourced, organic options is the right decision. Clarified butter (ghee) is also an excellent choice.

Nuts and Seeds

Almonds, walnuts, chia seeds are excellent sources of healthy fats with relatively low carbs. They are the best option when you feel the need for a snack. Be careful to not overeat though! It's very easy to eat too much and throw your Calorie counts off!

Oils

Oils are one of the worst offenders when it comes to chemical processing. Extra refined, frying oil, which is almost as clear as water is one of the worst things you can choose to consume.

Instead, choose whole oils like olive oil, coconut oil, almond oil, mustard oil and avocado oil. When purchasing these, make sure they are either virgin or cold pressed. You will find options these days for something called olive pomace oil. This is marketed as olive oil and is far cheaper than regular extra virgin olive oil. Stay away from it though since it is chemically treated and is just a marketing gimmick.

Cooking with these oils does take some getting used to since they tend to smoke at lower temperatures compared to refined oils. Also they do have a stronger taste due to their untarnished nature.

Low Carb Vegetables

On the keto diet you should avoid starchy, high carb vegetables like the following

- Tubers
- Carrots
- Beets
- Corn
- Green Peas
- Parsnips
- Sweet potato

- Pumpkin
- Yams

Instead, low carb options like the ones below

- Onions
- Peppers
- Tomatoes
- Spinach
- Kale
- Asparagus
- Broccoli
- Salad Greens
- Cucumber

While technically a fruit, the avocado belongs here. If the keto diet had to have a face, it would have to be the avocado's. Have it raw, as guacamole or as part of a salad, this fatty fruit has it all.

Miscellaneous

Condiments are a sneaky way to inadvertently cheat on the keto diet. Ketchup, mustard and the like are permissible as is salt and pepper. The thing you want to look out for is the sugar content of these condiments.

So a full fat ranch dressing might sound keto friendly but a store-bought item will almost invariably have a high amount of sugar in it. This is unlikely to be naturally-occurring sugar so stay away from it.

Artificial sweeteners can be used such as stevia, xylitol and sorbitol. While not a great idea, having some occasionally is perfectly fine. Coffee and tea are perfectly fine as long as they are consumed black and preferably unsweetened. Adding dairy to it will improve the keto-friendliness of it.

If you're a chocolate lover, dark chocolate is a wonderful option. Make sure to consume something with more than 80% cocoa though and organic if possible.

This concludes the list of permissible things to eat. As you can see there are many options and there's no real need to restrict yourself in any way. The key thing to keep in mind is that moderation in everything is key. Yes, you can consume cream and butter but this does not give you the license to down a full tub of it. Excess of anything is harmful and you need to maintain a caloric deficit, even on the keto diet, to lose fat.

Vegans might be panicking at this point because there don't seem to be many protein sources available. Indeed, meat is out of the question and the usual vegan protein sources like chickpeas and legumes are not compatible. There is a solution for this.

Among whole food, your protein choices are low to be honest. The best, perhaps only, keto sources of protein are:

- Seitan
- Tempeh
- Tofu

That's not much of a list. The best thing to do is to supplement using a vegan protein powder. Remember that going vegan is a great choice but you do need to put in some work to get the benefits. Do not give in to the temptation to consume less protein since it is absolutely essential you eat enough depending on your lifestyle goals.

Let us now look at the foods you ought to avoid on the keto diet.

Foods to Avoid

While we're clear on the fact that processed foods ought to be avoided, it still bears fruit to run through the list of foods you should not be eating. There will be some foods which you are used to eating which will not make the cut. Some of these might surprise you.

Sugary Foods

Sodas, fruit juices, ice cream, candy, chocolate cake, unless they happen to be keto versions, all fall under this category. This seems like a lot to give up, especially if you have a sweet tooth. Dark chocolate is the only substitute you have for this category and with discipline, you will find that you don't miss these foods anymore.

Grains

All grains like rice, wheat, barley, buckwheat and bulgur are to be avoided. You can substitute this with high protein grains like quinoa but you need to be aware of the amount of carbs you're consuming.

Fruits contain a high amount of naturally occurring sugar. While they are not unhealthy per se, given the presence of sugar, they do tend to increase the amount of glucose produced upon consumption. This, of course, interrupts the process of ketosis.

You can consume berries like strawberries, blueberries and raspberries.

Beans and Legumes

Legumes and beans are a great vegan source of protein but given the carb ratio in them, they are not suitable for a ketogenic diet. As detailed above though, there are ways to substitute for them successfully.

Tubers

Generally speaking, any starchy or root vegetable is not suited for the keto diet. So potatoes, sweet potatoes, turnips, beets, carrots and the vegetables listed in the list of starchy foods are out.

You can consume veggies like leafy greens, tomatoes, onions, cauliflower, cabbage, peppers, broccoli, kale etc.

Alcohol

This one should go without saying but alcohol should be minimized on the keto diet. Sticking to clear liquors which are have an alcohol content of over 40% will not throw you out of ketosis. Examples of this are vodka, whiskey, gin and scotch. The real issue with alcohol is the decreased consciousness and hunger pangs it brings and after a few drinks you might not be so inclined to stay disciplined when faced with a pizza. Also, almost all commercially available alcohol contains either added sugar or corn syrup. While the quantities are not large, much like saturated fat as explained previously, minimizing alcohol is the best way forward.

This list of foods to avoid tends to produce an adverse reaction. After all, a non-sugar, non-alcohol consuming existence does tend to be a bit boring. Well, fear not. As we'll see in the chapter dealing with meal plan design, there is a way to satisfy your cravings and still meet your goals.

As always, the message to keep in mind is moderation in everything. Now that we've finished with our in-depth look at the basics of the keto diet, let's now look at the different types of keto diets you can adapt based on your lifestyle goals.

Chapter 3: Types of Ketogenic Diets

Your lifestyle goals largely dictate your diet and exercise plan. It isn't enough to simply say "I want to lose fat". You also need to define what activity level you wish to carry out to achieve your goals.

You see, losing fat isn't just for the obese. You can be a perfectly healthy individual but wish to shed a few pounds of fat. The keto diet will help you do this in a healthy and controlled manner. Depending on your activity level, there are four options you could follow:

- The Standard Ketogenic Diet
- The High Protein Ketogenic Diet
- The Cyclical Ketogenic Diet
- The Targeted Ketogenic Diet

We'll go over them one by one starting with the standard diet. Before we dive in though, please keep in mind, when starting out it is a good idea to keep track of your macros.

This means, you track the carbs, fat and protein you're consuming. Once you're following the diet for a few weeks, you will gain an idea of roughly how much you're eating and whether this is correct or not. Also, all these diet principles apply equally to vegans so there's no additional advice or actions you need to take.

The Standard Ketogenic Diet

This is the boilerplate diet that fits almost everyone out there. This diet follows the rules laid out in the previous chapter, that is, low carbs and high fat. Whether you choose to follow this diet or not depends on your activity level.

Activity Level and Macros

For those who perform moderately intense activities like cycling, jogging, playing sports as recreation 2-3 times per week or even train in the gym 3-4 times per week, the standard diet (SKD) is ideal.

Now, estimating your activity level is a tricky thing. If you're a beginner you will almost always overestimate this. If you tend to perform high-intensity exercises (which we will cover later in detail), the standard diet isn't for you. This diet is excellent for those looking to shed a few pounds of fat and generally get into good shape.

The SKD is ideal if your exercise consists mostly of aerobic exercise like running, biking and other activities which involve minimal weight training. When starting off, you will experience a performance dip. The reason for this is similar to why you will experience the keto "fog" when starting out: your body just hasn't adjusted as yet.

Now on the SKD, you want to maintain the following macro ratio (macro refers to macronutrients, that is, proteins, carbs and fat). You need to eat at least 0.7-0.8 grams of protein for every pound of body weight. Next, you need to eat a maximum of 30 grams of carbs. The rest of your Calories should come from fat. Let's look at an example to see how this calculation plays out. First let's list our assumptions:

1. *Weight in pounds= 180*

2. *Target caloric intake= 2200 kcal*

Now let's assume we decide to eat 0.8 grams of protein per pound of body weight per day. Using the table in the first chapter (where the Calories per gram for the macros was listed), we can calculate the following:

3. *Amount of protein eaten in grams= 180*0.8= 144 grams*

4. *Calories from protein= 144*4= 576 kcal*

Next, we know the amount of carbs we're restricting ourselves to. It is recommended to begin with 30g and then reduce after a month or so, once you feel comfortable.

5. *Amount of carbs eaten in grams= 30*

6. *Calories from carbs (using the same table)= 30*4=120 kcal*

7. *Total calories from protein and carbs= 576+120= 696 kcal*

Given our caloric intake target of 2200 kcal, we now can see that we need to provide 1504 kcal from fat. (points 2-7)

Referring to the same table in chapter 1, we know that each gram of fat yields 9 kcal. So to generate 1504 kcal we need to eat:

8. *Grams of fat to consume per day= 1504/9= 167 g*

Thus our final macros are the following: 144g protein, 30g carbs and 167 g fat for a total of 2200 kcal per day.

This is how straightforward it is to calculate your macros. As you can see, once you get past the confusion and just stick to the basics, knowing what to eat and how much becomes a very simple task. It is these calculations upon which you will base your meals and diet plans.

Caloric Deficit

Now you might be wondering how we arrived at the figure of 2200 kcal in the first place? In other words, how do you determine how many Calories you need to eat in the first place? The answer lies in understanding a term called the BMR or Basal Metabolic Rate.

The BMR is the measure of how much energy a person expends on a given day given their activity level. This number is expressed in kcal and depends on the person's sex, age, height, weight and activity level. The activity level is the only wild card in all of this so it's better to underestimate how active you are when you're starting off.

There are a number of calculators online where you simply input these numbers and you receive your BMR. Now this number is the amount of calories you need to eat to maintain your current physical state. After all this is the amount of energy you expend daily. So if you eat this amount, you will maintain. This caloric level is called the maintenance level (clever, isn't it?).

If you wish to lose fat, you need to maintain a healthy caloric deficit as previously explained. So how much of a deficit is healthy? Roughly speaking, a 500 kcal deficit is considered healthy. The reason is this: over a 7 day period, maintaining a 500 kcal deficit results in an overall deficit of 500*7= 3500 kcal. This is how much you need to shed one pound of body fat. So at this rate, you will be shedding one pound per week and 4 pounds per month and so on.

Losing weight at a rate greater than this is not recommended for beginners. If you're experienced, you probably don't need to read all of this to begin with.

This is how you safely lose weight in a healthy manner and ensure you are not losing any muscle. We will discuss tracking progress and gains in a later chapter. For now, remember this simple process:

- Calculate BMR (via online calculators)
- Subtract 500 kcal from it. This is how much you need to eat per day
- Eat 0.8 grams of protein per pound of body weight per day. Calculate kcal from protein
- Eat 30 grams of carbs per day. Calculate kcal from carbs
- Add numbers in steps 2 and 3. Subtract this sum from the number in step 2.
- Divide the resulting number by 9 to determine grams of fat you need to eat per day.
- Track all metrics and adjust as required (discussed in later chapters)

The only thing left to do is determine your food list and your exercise plan. These will be covered in chapters ahead so don't worry. The aim here is to slowly build your knowledge and comfort level as opposed to overloading you with information.

Next, let us look at the high protein keto diet (HPKD).

The High Protein Ketogenic Diet

The high protein diet is quite similar to the SKD except for one thing. The amount of protein you'll be eating is increased. It is very important to understand when to use this diet and its aims. It all starts with delving into why you would even want to increase protein in the first place.

Protein and Muscle

As we saw in the first chapter where we covered the basics of nutrition, proteins are the building blocks of our muscles. Our muscles are literally made of amino acids which is the same stuff proteins are made of. Hence, the more protein you consume, the more food your muscles have. Right?

Well, not exactly. Our bodies aren't that easy to manipulate. The thing with protein is that beyond a certain amount, our bodies just can't process them anymore as intended and these excess proteins get converted into fat. Recall that our bodies have a priority list when it comes to converting food into either muscle or fat once it has converted food into whatever we need for energy.

If we've already fed our muscles, via a high amount of protein, there is no need to convert it into even more muscle and hence, the excess protein gets converted into fat. The trouble doesn't end there though.

Risks

Excess protein poses many health risks. The nitrogen prevalent in amino acids poses an especial risk to your liver. A 2002 study conducted amongst active athletes found a more concentrated urine as well as increased levels of blood urea nitrogen, which is a measure of kidney function1

[1](Cronkleton & Sullivan, 2019).

Other risks include weight gain, constipation ,diarrhea and a deficit of calcium. A side effect of this is also an increased risk of cancer, thanks to the copious amounts of meat one will presumably eat when following a very high protein diet.

So while the bro in your gym might preach protein, remember that like everything else, balance is essential.

---

[1] Cronkleton, E., & Sullivan, D. (2019). What Happens If You Eat Too Much Protein?. Retrieved from https://www.healthline.com/health/too-much-protein#recommended-daily-protein

Balance

So what is the healthy level of protein consumption? In adult males, this is a maximum of 1.5 grams per pound of body weight and in women it is 1.2 grams per pound of body weight. Anything above this is considered excessive.

When following the keto diet, given its emphasis on fat, if the additional calories you will consume from protein put you over your caloric limit, remove the excess by limiting the amount of carbs you eat, not fat.

Objective

This brings us back to our original point as to why you would want to eat a higher level of protein to begin with? Given that it helps build muscle, the answer is simple: If you wish to build more muscle, you increase the amount of protein you eat every day.

Now, if you want to build muscle, that is increase your body weight via more muscle, you cannot do this while maintaining a caloric deficit. Your body needs additional fuel to build things and it stands to reason it can't do anything if it doesn't have this excess fuel.

Thus, if your goal is solely to cut fat, an HPKD is not your solution. You need to either follow the SKD or one of the other two variations. If you're a beginner looking to add more muscle, the HPKD is a great choice since its straight forward like the SKD. The only difference is you maintain a caloric excess instead of a deficit.

Exercise and Excess

The amount of caloric excess you will need to maintain is 500 kcal. Much like how we saw with the SKD, this will result in your gaining 1 lb of muscle in body weight per week. The calculation of your macros is exactly the same as with the SKD.

This time instead of using 0.8 grams per pound of body weight, you use 1.2 to 1.5 grams of protein and calculate those calories. The amount of carbs remain the same and the remaining amount is sourced from fat.

Your exercise regimen plays an important role in building muscle. Following a plan of just cardiovascular exercises like cycling or aerobics will not build you muscle beyond a certain point. You will need to hit the weight room and follow a structured plan based on progressive overloading.

If that sounds like Greek to you, don't worry we'll cover all this in the chapters on building an exercise plan.

Tracking

With the HPKD, tracking is of even greater importance than the SKD. This is because with this diet plan, we're trying to achieve two objectives as opposed to just one. We're trying to build muscle while minimizing fat gain (as opposed to just losing fat with the SKD).

We'll cover this in greater detail later but for now keep in mind that you will have to track not just your food intake but also your exercise performance. You will initially suffer a dip in performance of course but once your body adapts, you should see an increase in strength as time progresses.

Generally, while looking to build muscle, cardio is not recommended since this inhibits muscle growth but rather than eliminate it completely, it is a good idea to merely minimize it. So if you usually do 30 minutes of cardio, reduce it to 10 and so on. HIIT or high-intensity cardio is not recommended on this diet, not because of a lack of performance, but simply because HIIT will burn your muscle along with the fat and this is contrary to your objectives.

Some people, no matter how hard they try, take longer to adapt to the keto diet. If you're one of these people, there is a solution for you. It is the CKD or Cyclical Ketogenic Diet.

The Cyclical Ketogenic Diet

As the name suggests, in this variation of the keto diet, you cycle in and out of ketosis. The idea is to get your body used to adapting by forcing it to switch between burning both glucose and fat as fuel.

This is also ideal for those who wish to test the waters when it comes to keto and are perhaps not ready to fully immerse themselves as yet. Now this is a good time to point out that the CKD is actually the most versatile of the ketogenic diet variations in that both beginners and more advanced dieters can implement this.

In the CKD, you will be consuming a high fat, low carb diet for five days of the week and for two days, you will switch to a moderate carb, moderate fat diet, that is, a normal diet. The idea is to replenish your glycogen stores in order to fuel your workouts or physical activities for the following week. If you're a beginner or someone who just isn't able to adapt to the SKD immediately or even after a week, this cycling helps ease you into the SKD gradually.

Given that these are two very different objectives, its well worth it to break down how the diet should work for both scenarios.

Gradual Easing

When starting out on the keto diet, if you don't perform and don't plan on performing any strenuous physical activity, the SKD is your best option. The drawback with this is the SKD adopts a sink or swim approach. If you're choosing to adopt the keto diet over a weekend, it might go like this: On Thursday, you have a regular amount of carbs. On Friday, all of a sudden, you're eating next to no carbs and huge amounts of fat.

Mentally and physically this is quite a change to make. Our bodies and minds are extremely resilient so you will be able to handle it without too many issues beyond the "fog" phase. For some though, this fog lasts longer or for whatever reason, they just take longer to adapt to the food they'll be eating now.

For example someone who has been consuming grains and legumes for their meals for over 20 years, suddenly giving this up will not be easy. They will feel the need to have something filling in their meals, that is, something that replicates the full feeling grains give them post meal times. If such people choose to eat salads, then there are two issues: 1) Salads don't give that full feeling and 2) They might 32not be able to digest raw vegetables easily leading to digestive issues.

For such people, CKD makes sense since it allows them to mentally and physically ease into the diet.

Goals

The first week after trying and failing to adopt the SKD, you could start the CKD. It is a good idea to keep your carb consuming days back to back, preferably towards the end of the week. You can have one of these days coincide with your cheat day, a concept we'll talk about when we look at the process of designing a meal plan. Remember, throughout all of this, you will be maintaining a caloric deficit.

During the two days, you will be consuming carbs, aim for the following when calculating your macros.

- Keep the protein level the same as you usually would
- Aim to eat 20% of your Calories from fat

That's all there is to it. So you will need to calculate your macros for these two days and figure out what you need to eat in what quantity. The period after you eat your carbs is more important when it comes to ensuring you progress towards your goals. You should aim to enter ketosis as soon as possible once you've finished your carb loading days.

The best way to do this is on the day following your second carb day, eat almost no carbs or 10g at the most. This forces your body to adapt and start burning fat for fuel. It also hastens the onset of ketosis and gets your body used to the fact that it needs to adapt fast and change the way it derives fuel.

Ideally, you don't want to stretch this cyclical period out to more than a month. It's easy to get comfortable doing this but remember the aim is to eventually move onto the SKD. Always keep this in mind when following the CKD.

Now, if you're someone who's more experienced with dieting and are used to performing high-intensity exercises, the CKD works for you as well. Let's see how.

Performance Oriented CKD

The idea of the carb loading that occurs as a part of CKD is to replenish your glycogen stores to fuel your workouts. This way you can continue to make gains in the gym while cutting fat and getting all the benefits of the keto diet. The other advantage of the CKD is that your body is not being deprived of carbs for long periods, as it would be with the SKD, and this assists your recovery and overall health.

When designing the schedule, you don't need to over think the times your carb loading days need to occur. The usual practice is to have them back to back on your weekly workout schedule. If you workout alternate days, you can have the first day on a workout day and second on a rest day or the other way around. The only scenarios to avoid are to have both days fall on rest days or have the day following the second day be a rest day.

This way you get the full benefit of carbs for muscle building and the benefits of the SKD during the remaining days. There are some things you will need to take into consideration though.

Macro Ratios

On your first loading day, your macro ratio should be 70% carbs, 20% proteins, and 10% fats. This, as you can see, is the exact opposite of the SKD. On the second carb loading day, change your ratio to 60% carbs, 25% proteins and 15% fat. In other words, you eat slightly fewer carbs and a little more protein and fat on the second day.

Opinion is divided as to when the carbs ought to be consumed. Conventional wisdom tells us that carbs are good for muscle growth and naturally, consuming them post workout seems ideal. However, there is also a branch of thought which proposes that carbs post workout may actually be hindering performance. As with all things nutrition, all these highlights is how much we still don't know how our bodies work.

Here's the best way to tackle this: On the first day, eat your carbs pre and post workout in whatever ratio you feel comfortable with. Go with whatever is the easiest and most comfortable for you. On the second day, your priority should be to get back into ketosis as soon as possible. Hence, consume carbs only pre-workout.

Which Carbs?

Not all carbs are created equal. Whether you're executing the CKD as a beginner or as an intermediate, it is essential for you to pick the right type of carbs for your nutrition. As a beginner, it is ideal for you to pick low GI carbs on your loading days. For the intermediates out there, pick a low GI carb on the first day and high GI carbs on the second day.

What is GI some of you might be wondering? Well, GI stands for glycemic index. This index which runs from 0-100 is a measure of the rapidity with which carb is digested and metabolized. Foods which rank high on the GI scale tend to get metabolized faster and result in a spike in blood sugar levels followed by a subsequent drop. Slower burning carbs of lower GI carbs produce a more even distribution and lesser spikes.

While high GI carbs by themselves sound bad, remember this applies for carbs eaten in significant quantities over a period of time. On the keto diet, you're not consuming anywhere near enough. However, to be on the safe side it's better to stick to low GI carbs. Examples of this include sweet potatoes, lentils and soy products.

Ketosis

You need to aim to get back into ketosis as soon as possible and this begins post workout on your second carb loading day. If you choose to have the second loading day on a rest day, no matter, aim to finish your carbs quota by early evening. Following this, you need to begin the process of hastening ketosis as much as possible.

This begins with a fasted workout the next morning. Ideally, this will be a long HIIT workout or a strength training workout followed by a small HIIT session. Make sure you supplement with BCAA prior to working out or else you will lose muscle. BCAA means BCAA, not protein powder or creatine. You need to fuel your muscles directly and as quickly as possible prior to workout.

Also fasted means no coffee or juice or anything. Just water and fat burner supplement should you need one and you're good to go. This regime forces your body to burn any excess glycogen it might have from the previous two days and to start using fat as fuel, that is, ketosis.

It is also a good idea to reduce the number of carbs you consume on this day to 10 grams to further emphasize the state of ketosis.

Goals and Results

It pays to constantly keep your goals in mind with all this since there is a fair amount of tracking required. With this sort of cycling followed by high-intensity workouts, you will be changing your body composition. Therefore it doesn't make sense to be in a deficit. Your aim should instead be maintenance. You can experiment with a slight deficit of say 250kcal per day but it might be too strenuous, especially for your post carb loading early morning workout.

Sticking to this religiously will recompose your lean body mass and fat percentage. Due to the cycling occurring, it is a good idea to purchase ketone testing strips, either via blood tests or urine to ensure you're entering ketosis as planned following your loading days.

Consistency

As mentioned previously the keto diet is not a magic bullet. The key is consistency and repeated action. Best results are obtained over a period of at least 90 days. This is when physical changes will be apparent and you'll be able to see them in the mirror.

Ultimately staying disciplined will help you achieve your goals than any diet out there. It will be difficult to stay in a caloric deficit for example for very long but if you remain mentally strong you will see your efforts bear fruit.

The CKD is a versatile option but sometimes, it just becomes a little too cumbersome. Calculating and tacking your different macro levels might seem like too much work for too little payoff. This is where the Targeted Ketogenic Diet or TKD comes in.

The Targeted Ketogenic Diet

One of the drawbacks with the CKD is that it requires you to step out of ketosis and re-enter. While the body is more than capable of handling this, mentally this does become taxing over longer periods of time. Over and above this, if you have cheat meals as most people do, you will find it difficult to schedule this along with your loading days and with the wrong schedule, you will find yourself out of ketosis quite a lot.

Naturally, if this happens a lot, you won't be receiving the full benefit of switching to a keto diet in the first place. This is where the TKD helps.

Precise Loading

The TKD functions on the same premise as the CKD, except the carb loading period is squeezed into a window right before your workout. The amount of carbs you eat is also tightly controlled. The idea is that the carbs help fuel your workout and performance and ideally, they glucose from the carbs will be exhausted within that time period, leaving you free to slip back into ketosis right after.

Reality is rarely this clean but the idea works more often than not. Again, the TKD is a diet for someone who performs high-intensity exercises or activities. If you're a beginner looking to lose fat, the SKD is your best bet.

Timing

To execute the TKD all you need to do is consume carbs around an hour prior to your workout. The amount of carbs consumed should be around 30 grams and not more than this. Also, needless to say, these carbs should be consumed only pre-workout, not post workout.

Your post-workout meal and nutrition are based on regular keto diet principles, that is high fat and low carb. Usually, you will find yourself out of ketosis for a few hours post workout but after that time period, it will restart. If you find yourself out of ketosis for extended periods for whatever reason, work out the next day on an empty stomach, with adequate BCAA supplementation, and you'll find yourself back in ketosis soon.

If this is a regular occurrence, there's something going wrong in your nutrition which bears examining.

High and Low GI

For your pre-workout carb load, you want to be consuming high GI carbs. This is because you need something to fuel you up quickly. A lower GI carb will not give you enough glucose in time for your workout, not to mention delay your ketosis onset.

You should also keep in mind that carb loading is not a license for you to binge and eat all sorts of junk. Very often, there is a mistaken belief that since you'll be burning everything anyway, you could just eat whatever you want. You still have to follow proper nutrition rules, that is, stay away from processed foods or foods high in sugar.

Sugary food and drink will seem like the best option for a pre-workout load since they provide instant energy. The long term effects of processed sugar are damaging though and you ought to stay away from it.

Post Workout

Your post-workout nutrition should follow regular keto diet rules. A protein shake is the best option if you cannot have a heavy meal immediately.

This concludes our look at the different types of keto diets. As you can see there is an option available for everyone, no matter where on the experience scale you fall. The most important thing to remember is that your diet needs to be allied to your activity level.

We'll be looking at the activity levels and the various workout you can fit into them later in the book. For now though, it is important we look at one of the most overlooked areas of dieting: supplementation.

Chapter 4: Supplements

Supplements get a bad rep mostly due to ignorance and other commercial factors. Say the word supplement and most people immediately think of steroids. While steroids are a form of supplement, they are far removed from the world of regular supplements. It's a bit like saying all fish in the ocean are like sharks and that you should avoid swimming near all of them.

On the keto diet, it is not strictly necessary for you to supplement. They do help though. For vegans, it is absolutely necessary since there just aren't enough protein options out there. Another reason to supplement is to help fuel your workouts. You see, the best way to lose fat is to work out in a fasted state. Now, as you can imagine, it is pretty difficult to get going on an empty stomach. You simply cannot do this without the help of supplements.

Supplements have come a long way since the early days when almost everything was some sort of steroid. While they are completely safe, you still ought to remember they are called supplements for a reason. They merely assist you in your diet. They are not a diet in and as of themselves. Given the volume of them in the market, it can be difficult to remember this. Whole food is still your best bet to achieve all your nutritional goals.

Let us now look at some of the most useful supplements and some other not so useful ones which are simply a drain on your wallet for all purposes. All of these are vegan friendly and in the case of protein powder, vegan friendly options are available as noted.

Useful Supplements

It is not necessary for you to purchase these supplements but they are nice to have. The ones which are absolutely necessary for certain people, for example, vegans, will be highlighted clearly.

Multivitamins

These are the most popular supplements taken regularly by people. The reality, however, is that their degree of helpfulness is still not fully clear. While we do know that a deficiency of vitamins is bad for our immune system and that it increases our risk of heart disease and other undesirable conditions, we still don't know whether ingesting them in a pill form is as effective as it ought to be. The consensus is that consuming them via whole food is the best but it is extremely difficult and counterproductive to track vitamin consumption like macros. Hence, everyone seems to agree that doing something is better than nothing so pills are the best option we have as of now.

Some of the most common deficiencies found are for Vitamin D and Vitamin B12. Vitamin D, as most of you may know, is produced via exposure to sunlight. This is an especial problem for people in countries which suffer from extended winters. In such cases, a specialized Vitamin D supplement is recommended along with a general multivitamin.

B12 is often found deficient in vegans and vegetarians since this is found exclusively in animal products. Needless to say, if you're a vegan living in Norway, your first purchase ought to be a multivitamin supplement. If you're over the age of 50, multivitamins are a must for you, whether you're on the keto diet or not.

Creatine

Creatine is a bit controversial as a supplement. You see, there's no doubt that it does help stimulate muscle growth. The issue is whether you actually need it if you're able to more than eat whole food. Some studies report the gains to be marginal and some indicate that creatine is often a direct stimulant. One wonders why there's so much confusion around nutrition!

When it comes to the keto diet, supplementing creatine is a choice that depends on your goals. If you're looking to build muscle then adding creatine to your diet is worth it. If you're looking to cut fat or recompose your physique then on a keto diet creatine probably isn't going to make a significant difference. It will have an effect no doubt but since your goal is not to build muscle, it might not be the most effective use of it.

As a beginner, you really don't need creatine. In fact, at this stage, you're better off with a few supplements. This is because, at a beginner's stage, almost anything you do will make a huge difference. Strength gains in the gym will give you a much better physique than creatine ever will. So focus on exercising well and building up your expertise in that regard.

If you're performing high-intensity activities with the goal of building muscle as part of your workout routine then creatine is a perfect choice. Combined with whey protein, creatine will give you major performance gains and will also reduce your need to load on high GI carbs.

Omega 3

Here's a fun fact: Our brain's composition is 40% DHA which is an omega 3 fatty acid. If you aren't eating fatty fish every week, you're one of the many people who are deficient in this. Fish oil is the most well-known supplement for omega 3 with the capsules containing doses of both EPA and DHA, another omega 3 acid.

Recommended intake is 250-500 mg per day. Depending on the size of the capsule, your dosage will vary. This supplement is necessary no matter which diet you follow.

Vegans need not worry, there are readily available plant sources for omega 3. It must be said, however, that plant sources aren't as rich compared to fish and you will have to consume a lot more of them in order to meet your requirement. Chia seeds, flax seeds, walnuts, and hemp seeds are excellent plant-based sources. Flax seeds also double as an excellent fiber supplement which we'll be looking at next, so they are a win-win.

The best way to meet this requirement would be to mix the powder of these seeds into your meals throughout the day as opposed to setting aside a particular time to eat it.

Fiber

On a high protein, high-fat diet, you will suffer from a lack of fiber. There's no getting away from it. One way of increasing the amount of fiber in your diet is to eat a lot of leafy green vegetables like lettuce, cabbage and spinach.

However, you are not a rabbit and there's only so much lettuce you can eat. A fiber supplement is essential to prevent constipation and other nasty surprises. For a change, the vegans have it easier here since the greater amount of plant-based foods their diet has, the overall fiber content will be higher. For meat eaters, any off the shelf fiber supplement will more than do the job, there's no need to get creative with this.

Whey and Casein Protein

Whey and casein protein are both found in milk. However, with dairy being off limits, the best way to supplement this, if needed, is to consume protein powder. You will usually see whey powder and casein powder being sold separately and lots of articles online about how one is better than the other. Let's break this down a little.

The only difference between the two you need to be aware of is that whey is a fast acting protein and casein is a slow acting one. This means whey behaves much like a high GI carb and immediately gives you the boost you need while casein is released slower into the bloodstream. Both have their advantages. Whey gives you an instant performance boost and is excellent as a pre-workout shake. Casein is useful because it provides a steady, sustained stream of protein for your muscles over a longer period, especially relevant if you consume it before going to bed.

If you're vegan, a vegan whey protein powder is absolutely essential, as mentioned previously. Don't try to second guess this and think you can eat more tofu or something, just go buy one. The amount you consume will be dictated by your macro calculations.

For the rest, it really depends on your goals and whether you're comfortable eating more or less whole food. If you're looking to build muscle, then a casein protein powder is a good idea since it will minimize muscle breakdown overnight and aid recovery. If you're trying to lose fat, this is much like creatine and you can take a call either way.

BCAA

Branch chain amino acids or BCAA is something we've touched upon previously when talking about the CKD and TKD. If you're on the SKD you really don't need this. For those on the CKD or TKD, this is absolutely essential for your morning fasted workouts.

Those on the SKD might want to consider this if they wish to workout fasted. This is not something recommended for beginners, even though it results in the fastest fat loss since it takes a lot of mental strength to do this. You won't see too many experienced gym rats training fasted unless they absolutely have to.

There are a lot of recent studies being done recently which are rethinking the way BCAAs work and whether they are useful or not. At this point there haven't been enough conclusions to be statistically significant so for now, we will just rely on the experience of trainers over the years. This is something to watch out for, however.

So to summarize, consuming around 10g BCAA prior to your fasted workout and have a protein shake post workout. You don't really need BCAA if you're not training fasted.

Fat Burner

This is another supplement you need to take only if you're working out fasted. Fat burners don't actually burn fat, they're just branded that way. What they do is they give you a burst of energy which propels you to workout harder than you usually would and thus, burn more Calories.

If you feel especially lethargic in the mornings, then consider supplementing some fat burner. If not, leave it be. A cup of coffee without milk works just as well.

Mineral Tablets

Minerals like zinc, calcium, and magnesium serve major purposes when it comes to your bodily functions. Supplementing them is always a good idea, especially zinc, which will help aid your recovery post workout. The best way of ingesting them, as mentioned previously, is via whole food. As long as you ensure your diet is well balanced and has healthy amounts of leafy greens you will almost certainly be consuming the required quantities of minerals.

In addition, on the keto diet, you will experience a lot of water loss and with that comes a loss of electrolytes like sodium, magnesium, potassium and calcium. You will need to keep track of your water intake and be on the lookout for signs of dehydration like headaches, decreased performance and activity levels.

Your diet should be balanced enough to cover all your needs if you consume food as directed in this book but its recommended you supplement with tablets as well to reduce the risk of deficiencies..

Supplements You Don't Need

The market is awash with stuff you don't need unless you're a bodybuilder, and even they only need steroids. So this list is of stuff you really need not pay any attention to, even if you're looking to build muscle or optimize your workouts.

Some of them are actually good but are only useful marginally while some are just flat out marketing gimmicks.

Conjugated Linoleic Acid

CLA is one of those magic pills come true. Once consumed it burns off all fat and stimulates muscle growth. CLA is a fat that is mostly found in meat and dairy.

All of the above is 100% true....for rodents. That's right! CLA was initially tested on rodents and the results were hugely encouraging. Unfortunately, tests done on humans are completely inconclusive since, surprise, the human body is just a tad more complex than a rat's.

Those spammy ads you see promising a magic pill are usually CLA mixed with some other junk. Needless to say, you really don't need this.

Glutamine

This one is a staple at any fitness store and online health store. Sadly, many trainers have drunk the kool-aid on this one. The reasoning for glutamine being necessary is sound enough.

Patients suffering heave burn injuries or muscle loss via disease are treated with doses of glutamine. This is an amino acid and patients experience remarkable recovery in their musculature. However, glutamine only seems to work when the level of muscle loss is excessive.

No matter how much of a beast you are in the gym, you simply will not suffer the level of muscle loss necessary to make glutamine useful.

Garcinia Cambogia

This one is a popular "mystery herb" which promises extreme fat loss via a "weird" trick. The reality is you're just eating something that tastes funny and has an exotic name.

There have not been any studies showing the effectiveness of this so stay away from it.

Green Coffee Bean Extract

Yet another magical fat burner. The reason this one deserves a place on this list, instead of the other one despite being a fat burner, is the eternal promise of the green coffee bean as if its something special.

As explained previously, fat burners are not meant to burn fat. They just give you a shot of energy and off you go to the gym. This works much the same way but the green coffee bean part is used to justify higher prices.

As mentioned in the previous section on fat burners, a cup of black coffee works just as well prior to a fasted workout.

Deer Antler Spray

You can't be serious...

Nitric Oxide

This is actually a well-meaning supplement but just not that effective or even necessary when it comes down to it.

Nitric Oxide is a necessary chemical which aids in our overall well being and health. Its just that if you follow a good diet, like the keto diet, and have your share of vegetables, you're probably getting all the nitric oxide you need.

So you really don't need this in pill form.

Calcium

Yet another big one! Calcium is often marketed as being necessary for our bones and for the longest time, this was believed to be true. While it is correct that our bones are made of calcium, it does not follow that ingesting calcium in a pill form is going to aid bone strength.

In fact, many nutritionists and doctors have proposed that excessive calcium supplementation leads to calcification of our bones. In short, this is not something you want.

Specialized Protein

You'll often see supplements like beef protein or chicken protein or some such. If you're vegan, it makes sense to purchase a vegan protein powder but even in this case, a pill doesn't make sense.

For the non-vegans, a regular whey or casein protein supplement does the job, you really don't need to worry about the superiority of beef protein versus turkey or chicken. If you really are fanatical about this, go eat a steak.

Stay away from the powders and pills.

This concludes our look at the world of supplements. As you can see, there are many options but the thing to remember above all else is that they are not strictly required (with a few exceptions) unless there are special conditions or goals you have. Above all else, this should guide your decision making.

Chapter 5: Exercise and Workouts

Much like nutrition and our bodies' reaction to it, exercise and its role is something that is often filled with pseudoscience and hearsay. Just like diets, there are a number of options to choose from and it always seems like adopting one approach means sacrificing another. Most people end up losing perspective of the basic rule of exercise which is: just do something.

You need to do something every day that helps you break a sweat. This is the true role of exercise. Specialized workouts exist only for athletes who operate a very specialized level. For over 95% of people, a general workout which follows basic principles does the job. As we did in the nutrition chapters of this book, we're going to go back to basics and look at the different categories into which all exercises fall into.

It is important to state this at this point: There is no such thing as "the best fat burning exercise". This is because fat loss depends almost entirely on nutrition. As mentioned previously, you can lose weight without exercise but it's better not to. All exercise will help you burn fat, some better than others. What matters most is that you're doing something so don't worry too much about missing out on some special routine's benefits by doing something else.

Types of Exercise

Broadly speaking exercise can be classified into categories depending on the nature of the exercise or based on the goals you want to achieve with the exercise. Let's first look at classifying them on the basis of nature.

In this method, we can divide all forms of exercise into aerobic and anaerobic exercise. The difference between the two all comes down to oxygen as we shall see.

Aerobic Exercise

In aerobic exercise, the heart pumps out oxygenated blood out to the muscles that are working. Put in a simpler way, running, cycling, swimming, dancing, hiking and the like when performed at a low intensity, that is, where you're going along at a decent pace but not sprinting, is aerobic exercise. When you hear people referring to cardio in the gym, this is what they mean. Aerobic exercise has a number of health benefits for both our breathing and cardiovascular systems as a whole.

You see, our heart is a muscle and its job is to pump oxygenated blood to all parts of our body. The lungs, when you inhale, provide this oxygen and as the oxygen is delivered to the heart, it pumps this out along with blood to our body in order for it to function. The stronger our heart is, the more it can pump on a single beat (which is simply the contraction and expansion process of the pump). This increased efficiency is a good thing as our heart needs to work less to produce greater results.

This is why, if you're unfit or don't exercise much, your resting heart rate will be higher than someone who exercises more. Your heart, if unfit, has to do a lot more work to perform at the same level as the person who exercises. This is also why at a lower level of physical exertion, compared to a person who is fitter, you run out of breath because your heart simply cannot keep up with your oxygen demands.

Aerobic exercise trains your lungs and your heart to pump oxygen more efficiently. As you exercise, your lungs are put to the test and their ability to take more air in and deliver the oxygen to the heart is tested. Once the oxygen is delivered, you are demanding a higher level of performance from your heart, via exercise, and the heart has to pump faster and more efficiently to meet your demands.

This oxygen once delivered to the muscles is used to burn fuel. As we saw previously, fuel is either glucose or fat and whichever is present is burned to fuel your muscles and produce performance. The thing about burning fat as fuel is that, being denser than glucose, it requires a greater amount of oxygen to burn. In turn, fat release a greater amount of energy, 9kcal per gram as opposed to 4 kcal per gram of glucose, as we saw in the very first chapter.

What all this means is that if you're on a keto diet and performing aerobic exercise, you're forcing your heart to pump more oxygen in order to burn fat. This trains your heart to be more efficient and it also ends up burning off your fat at a faster rate. As an aside, this is why what you eat matters more than how you exercise. Since all exercise produces the same effect on the heart, that is it needs to deliver oxygen to the muscles more efficiently, fat loss really comes down to this: is your body burning glucose or fat? The more fat it burns, the leaner you become. Hence, remove the glucose and force your body to burn the fat. The removal of glucose is entirely down to your diet.

Aerobic exercise also forces your muscles to consume the oxygen delivered to them more efficiently. The reason you get better at exercising the more you do it because your muscles have adapted to consuming oxygen and fuel more efficiently. This consumption is referred to as VO2. It is expressed in units of ml/kg per minute. Your body's VO2 max is the optimum rate at which your muscles can effectively utilize what is delivered to them. Keep this term in mind since we'll revisit it in the section on anaerobic exercise.

Aerobic exercise also has great psychological effects by helping reduce anxiety and depression. IN short, aerobic exercise simply makes you feel good!

So all of this sounds great so far and to be frank it is mostly so. There are some drawbacks to aerobic exercise from the perspective of someone who's looking at building all round health. Aerobic exercise is the best way to build your endurance, that is your body's ability to enhance its VO2. It is not a great way to build strength, that is, to increase the size of your muscles.

The more aerobic exercise you do, the more your body adapts. Your muscles adapt into the form best suited to consume oxygen as efficiently and as quickly as possible in order to fuel you for longer. This adaptation results in a base level of strength or a minimum required level of strength, beyond which the muscles prioritize burning fuel more efficiently. This is why, if you watch the Olympics, you will notice the physique of long-distance athletes is quite frail. Some of them, if they're reasonably tall, appear almost emaciated. Marathon runners tend to have a similar, slim physique. While such athletes have an incredible cardiovascular ability, being able to perform at high speed over incredibly long distances, they are not quite barometers of strength.

As an everyday Joe, you're probably more concerned with looking good than achieving God-like levels of cardio performance. Thus while it pays to engage in aerobic exercise, you need to supplement it with anaerobic exercise as well.

Anaerobic Exercise

Anaerobic exercise, as the name suggests, refers to exercises performed where your body lacks oxygen or where your heart simply is able to deliver oxygen fast enough to your muscles. This sounds less like anaerobic and more like "inducing death" but this is actually a great way to train your heart and muscles.

Anaerobic exercises are performed at very high intensity since the aim is to deplete oxygen stores. Almost any aerobic activity can be made anaerobic by performing it faster. For example, if you were to cycle on a mountainous road at a pace more appropriate for the Tour de France, you're engaging in anaerobic exercise. Cycling in a park at a leisurely pace would be aerobic exercise.

So why is anaerobic exercise good for you? You see, as oxygen stores deplete, your muscles are forced to look elsewhere for fuel sources. This forces them to burn their existing energy stores, which is usually accessed only in emergencies, and thus conditions your muscles to go longer and become stronger since their primary fuel source is cut off.

As you can imagine, this state of things doesn't last very long. Anaerobic exercise is performed in short, sharp burst of activity, as opposed to aerobic exercise which is performed at low intensity for a longer period of time. Using the example of the Olympics, the 10,000-meter race is an aerobic activity whereas the 100-meter sprint is anaerobic.

Contrast the physiques of Olympic sprinters with the long distance runners and you'll see the sort of results anaerobic exercise produces. Aside from this, there are other benefits too including high-intensity exercise in your routine. Your muscles will become stronger with anaerobic routines since they are forced to support you and perform despite a lack of oxygen. This forces them to adapt and the result is you gain a higher level of strength. In addition to this, your bones also become stronger and there is the usual psychological benefit as well.

The biggest benefit though is to your VO2 max which increases. In other words, your body's cardiovascular system as a whole becomes more efficient. Your lungs deliver oxygen to your heart faster, your heart becomes more efficient at pumping out oxygenated blood and your muscles learn to use every single unit of oxygen to burn fuel more efficiently. Thus your endurance level rises.

It must be noted that though your endurance improves, it will not reach the levels it can if employing aerobic exercise. Think of it this way: Usain Bolt, being as great as he is, is not winning any medals in the 10,000-meter race. In fact, it'll be quite an achievement if he even qualifies for the finals. His body is optimized to deliver energy in short sharp bursts, not at a constant rate over long periods.

This higher intensity is also ideal for fat loss, compared to aerobic exercise. Due to the strain produced in your body while performing anaerobic exercises, your body remains in fuel burning mode for far longer than it would be performing aerobic exercise. If you're on the keto diet, this is excellent news since you'll burn even more fat given the glycogen depletion you induce via your diet.

There are obvious drawbacks to anaerobic exercise though. Aside from a lower level of endurance and the mentally taxing nature of it, if performed over a long session, it will result in muscle depletion. This is because once the energy stored within your muscles are depleted, your body has no choice but to burn your muscles for energy. Thus it is extremely easy to overtrain if you're not keenly aware of your session times.

Anaerobic exercise is not a great option for beginners since its demanding nature requires you to have a base level of strength and endurance for it to be effective. In the beginning, you probably won't be able to even approach the intensity levels required. Thus, it is best, as a beginner, to perform aerobic exercises first and then gradually build up to anaerobic ones.

So this is the way to categorize exercises based on their physiological functions. The other way we can classify exercise is via our goals, that is, do we wish to maximize strength or endurance? On the surface, this seems to be the same as aerobic versus anaerobic exercise but strength training has a key element we haven't looked at as yet and that is weight training.

Weight training is an extremely versatile method and can be geared towards both aerobic and anaerobic. This topic is, however, the one most plagued by pseudoscience and misinformation. Given the extreme lack of clarity, it is a good idea to dive into the basics of weight training and examining how it can help you achieve goals in both the strength and endurance department. We will also look at things like sets and rep ranges and what range produces what type of results. If you have no idea what a set or a rep is, don't worry, this will all be covered shortly.

Weight Training Basics

Weight training, as mentioned previously, is an extremely versatile way to increase your strength and endurance. It bears mentioning at this point that, the best way of increasing your endurance is via aerobic exercise or cardio. When training with weights you will find that most endurance exercises are of the anaerobic, high-intensity kind. Let's first see how weight training can improve your strength.

Strength Training

If there's one workout philosophy that will benefit you the most, it is strength training. Simply put, as long as you eat right and train for strength, you will lose fat, build muscle and feel better. Even if you are female or vegan or whatever, this works for everyone. Simply put, the stronger you are, the easier everything is. Hopefully, that needs no explanation.

Secondly, one of the many benefits of strength training is the boost it gives your metabolism. The reason for this is that strength training affects something called EPOC or Excess Post-exercise Oxygen Consumption. This is the amount of oxygen your body needs to bring itself back to where it was prior to your workout. This recovery period can last for a while after your workout, depending on how strenuous it was, and while recovering your body continues to burn excess calories.

The more anaerobic your workout is, the greater the EPOC and the greater the number of calories you will burn post workout. Strength training is one of the best ways of achieving this due to the very nature of workouts. Here's what the American Council on Exercise has to say about this, via their website: (McCall, 2019)[1]

Strength training with compound, multijoint weightlifting exercises or doing a weightlifting circuit that alternates between upper- and lower-body movements places a greater demand on the involved muscles for ATP from the anaerobic pathways. Increased need for anaerobic ATP also creates a greater demand on the aerobic system to replenish that ATP during the rest intervals and the post-exercise recovery process. Heavy training loads or shorter recovery intervals increase the demand on the anaerobic energy pathways during exercise, which yields a greater EPOC effect during the post-exercise recovery period.[2]

---

[1] McCall, P. (2019). 7 Things to Know About Excess Post-exercise Oxygen Consumption (EPOC). Retrieved from https://www.acefitness.org/education-and-resources/professional/expert-articles/5008/7-things-to-know-about-excess-post-exercise-oxygen-consumption-epoc

[2] McCall, P. (2019). 7 Things to Know About Excess Post-exercise Oxygen

The same article(McCall, 2019) further points out:

In an extensive review of the research literature on EPOC, Bersheim and Bahr (2003) concluded that "studies in which similar estimated energy cost or similar exercising VO2 have been used to equate continuous aerobic exercise and intermittent resistance exercise, have indicated that resistance exercise produces a greater EPOC response." For example, one study found that when aerobic cycling (40 minutes at 80 percent Max HR), circuit weight training (4 sets/8 exercises/15 reps at 50 percent 1-RM) and heavy resistance exercise (3 sets/8 exercises at 80-90 percent 1-RM to exhaustion) were compared, heavy resistance exercise produced the biggest EPOC.[3]

Strength training also has been shown to help manage and improve the quality of life for people with the following diseases:

Consumption (EPOC). Retrieved from https://www.acefitness.org/education-and-resources/professional/expert-articles/5008/7-things-to-know-about-excess-post-exercise-oxygen-consumption-epoc

[3] McCall, P. (2019). 7 Things to Know About Excess Post-exercise Oxygen Consumption (EPOC). Retrieved from https://www.acefitness.org/education-and-resources/professional/expert-articles/5008/7-things-to-know-about-excess-post-exercise-oxygen-consumption-epoc

Osteoporosis

A study found that bone density increased even in elderly patients following a program of strength training (Veracity, 2019)[4].

From the article (Veracity, 2019):

Numerous studies demonstrate strength training's ability to increase bone mass, especially spinal bone mass. According to Keeton, a research study by Ontario's McMaster University found that a year-long strength training program increased the spinal bone mass of postmenopausal women by nine percent. Furthermore, women who do not participate in strength training actually experience a decrease in bone density.[5]

Parkinson's Disease

A study conducted at the University of Illinois at Chicago concluded that strength training significantly improved the motor skills of patients with Parkinson's disease("Long-term

---

[4] Veracity, D. (2019). Bone density sharply enhanced by weight training, even in the elderly. Retrieved from https://www.naturalnews.com/010528_bone_density_mineral.html

[5] Veracity, D. (2019). Bone density sharply enhanced by weight training, even in the elderly. Retrieved from https://www.naturalnews.com/010528_bone_density_mineral.html

weight training may benefit Parkinson's disease patients", 2019)

Lymphedema

A study carried out on breast cancer survivors concluded that strength training resulted in *"a decreased incidence of exacerbations of lymphedema, reduced symptoms, and increased strength"*(Schmitz et al., 2009).

Fibromyalgia: (Häkkinen A et al., 2001).

Cancer Survivors: (De Backer et al., 2007).

As should be evident by now, strength training's benefits go beyond mere physical changes.

Workouts

Strength training workouts tend to be of higher intensity but this doesn't mean you're running around all the time. It just means you'll be lifting close to your maximum effort every time you lift a weight. Getting started in strength training is easy. You simply do all the exercises listed below for the indicated sets and reps.

A rep stands for repetitions and is the number of times you will be lifting the weight. A set is simply one set of how many ever reps you choose to do together prior to resting. Strength training workouts usually have 5 sets of 5 reps for each exercise or 3X5 (3 sets of 5 reps).

So if you're going to squat 5X5, this means you squat 5 times then rest, then 5 times again and rest and repeat this three more times. In 3X5, you'll be squatting for 5 reps three separate times.

As for the list of exercises you need to do, there is a very small number. While the correct form for these exercises is beyond the scope of this book, you can find excellent videos and articles on how to execute them correctly. It is best to begin with an empty barbell and master your form before progressing further. The exercises you will need to do are:

1. Squats (back or front)
2. Overhead Barbell Press
3. Deadlift
4. Bench Press
5. Barbell Rows

That's it! You will not be doing all of these exercises at once in the same workout session. Instead, you will just perform the squat and rotate the other exercises around it for 3 days or 4 days per week.

There are many resources available online for you to design a strength training workout revolving around these five exercises. One of the benefits of strength training is that the workout is very simple to design and follow since there aren't many movements you're doing. They are also brutally effective since all these movements are total body workouts and thus burn the most calories which in turn means greater fat loss as your performance on them increases.

You might have heard of people complaining about injuries via strength and weight training. This is because all these exercises are technical in nature and you should always perform them with proper form. Getting injured by practicing poor form and blaming the exercise for being dangerous is a lot like driving down the wrong side of the road and blaming your car for the ensuing accident.

Women have special blocks to strength training, or training like a man, as many seem to think. Here's the deal: if you train like a man, you'll look like a goddess. There's no workout in this world that can make you look like a man unless you take an ungodly amount of steroids. Eat right and train hard and you'll look leaner and be stronger. Being strong does not mean having bulging muscles like a bodybuilder! Neither does it mean you'll look like the women in bodybuilding magazines. As mentioned earlier, looking like that requires you to ingest steroids and nothing in here calls for that.

Training for Shape

Weights can be used to tone your muscles and give them a desirable shape as well. While strength training focuses on building raw strength, there isn't much it does in the way of aesthetics beyond making you look leaner. In other words, you will not be able to have an 8 pack of abs via strength training alone. You will look fit but lack the definition you often see in images of celebrities and fitness models.

Some people are perfectly happy with this of course and there is no rule that says you need to look like a fitness model. There are some though who prefer to have a lot of definition in their muscles. Once you've built up your strength to an intermediate level, you can then begin to focus on toning your muscles and achieving a pleasing aesthetic look.

To do this you will have to perform what is called isolation exercises. While strength training focuses on total body movements, isolation movements are focused on just one portion of muscles, like the chest, shoulder, calves and so on.

Exercises for strength are done free, with just weight balanced on a barbell. Isolation exercises usually involve dumbells and machines. The number of sets is lower than on strength training exercises but the number of reps is higher, usually in the 8-12 range. So you will be performing sets of 3X12 or 2X15 even (3 sets of 12 reps and 2 sets of 15 reps).

Once you reach an appropriate level, you can cycle between strength training and higher rep training to ensure gains in both areas. The exercises that you can do under this sort of training are numerous, too numerous in fact to list out here, but even a simple search online will yield favorable results.

As for rotating, ideally, you want to perform one or two strength training exercises and then supplement them with the higher rep exercises. This will cause an increase in the number of days you have to go to the gym since you'll have to extend your strength training out to an extra day. However, combined with a cardio session at the end this is an excellent fat burning workout.

Cardio and Endurance Training

Cardiovascular training or simply cardio is relatively straight forward. There are two types of cardio, broadly speaking, steady state and high intensity. Steady state cardio is essentially aerobic exercise while HIIT is anaerobic. Again, aerobic and anaerobic exercise doesn't just involve cardio.

While starting out it is best to perform steady state cardio after your strength workouts. You don't need to overdo it, a period of 10-15 minutes is more than enough. Once your workouts rise in intensity, you'll find 10 minutes more than adequate.

You can choose to jog, cycle, swim or hop on the elliptical machine in your gym. Make sure to get your heart rate up to around to 50% of your maximum heart rate. You can calculate this by subtracting your age from 220. 50% of that resulting number is what you want to aim at in your cardio sessions.

Once you've built up a base standard of strength and endurance you can start experimenting with interval training or HIIT. HIIT stands for High-Intensity Interval Training and is an anaerobic form of exercise. HIIT combined with strength training will give you the maximum amount of fat loss possible.

It is, however, extremely taxing mentally when you first begin. The structure of a HIIT workout goes something like this. You exercise at full speed for an interval and then rest for an interval. You repeat this sequence over a period of 10-15 minutes. If you're doing HIIT at the end of your workout, its best to stick to just 10 minutes or else you'll risk muscle loss and excessive stress buildup.

The work and rest interval lengths are usually in a ratio of 1:2 when you begin. So if you work for one minute you rest for two. You need to really crank up your activity level and get your heart rate at least 80% of your maximum heart rate. This will be difficult to do at first so it's better to choose intervals of a minute which will allow you to build up to that level. Your aim should be to get there as fast as possible, not get there at the 58th second.

Once you have a measure of how soon you can get your heart rate up, you adjust your work interval length and rest interval accordingly and as you progress you shorten the rest interval until the ratio is inverted. That is, you'll be working twice as long as you rest. Another advanced option is to opt for Tabata intervals. Beginners to HIIT are cautioned against adopting this because of the issue of getting your heart rate up. Tabata intervals tend to be short and most beginners aren't used to the extreme activity levels HIIT demands.

Handling the mental stress is perhaps the toughest part of HIIT. The levels of exhaustion you will experience is unlike anything else due to the extreme demands being placed on you. As a rule of thumb, if you aren't completely exhausted, you're probably not pushing hard enough. As you can imagine, doing all this fasted (on CKD) is extremely taxing.

If you choose to do just HIIT, an optimal workout time limit is 20 minutes. You can choose just about any activity to perform be it cycling, sprinting or even hopping on the elliptical machine. Swimming is not recommended for obvious reasons unless its a shallow pool or you're an extremely good swimmer. You can perform HIIT using weights as well. A back squat or front squat with low weights will do the job but this is advisable only if you're extremely confident and proficient with your mechanics. The last thing you want to do is injure yourself.

The Ideal Workout

You might as well know this right off the bat: the ideal workout doesn't exist. The best workout to perform is one that challenges you to push your limits and more often than not leaves you energized at the end of it. There will be times when you will be exhausted but overall, if your workouts are pumping you up and improving your quality of life, then you're doing things correctly.

Most people expect instant results and when they don't see the changes in the mirror they get upset and lose motivation. As mentioned earlier it will take at least three months for physical changes to show up. Resist the temptation to chop and change due to thinking the grass is greener on the other side. Pick a workout routine that feels good and stick to it.

The more you keep things simple, the easier it will be for you to follow your routines. A lot of beginners tend to sabotage themselves by adopting new routines and adding and removing things all the time in the hope of getting better results. The reality is that fat loss and good fitness is simple and has been complicated thanks to erroneous knowledge and marketing.

Your body is not a snowflake so go ahead and test it rigorously. You'll be pleasantly surprised by the results you achieve.

Other Workouts

It isn't necessary for you to take up weight training of course. If you feel more comfortable running or swimming then feel free to do so. Just remember that adding muscle will help increase your performance in those activities too. At the very least, two days aimed at muscle building per week is a good idea. This way you get to do what you like and you're helping hasten your fat loss as well.

There are a lot of new training methods out there like Zumba these days which make for fun workouts. While these are great to partake in, remember that they don't build muscle beyond a certain point and if you stick only to them, you will hit a fat loss plateau and won't break past it because your body just doesn't have enough muscle to justify burning more fat.

The more muscle you have, the lesser the need for body fat so it is essential you focus on this as mentioned previously, at a minimum for 2 days per week.

Now that we've looked at training, let's combine this knowledge with what we know about the keto diet and see how you can marry the two together.'

Chapter 6: Training Plans

The type of training you choose to do will be dictated by the diet plan you choose to follow. If you're a beginner, for example, the SKD will fit you the best and as far as training goes, it's best to start off with something you're familiar with and comfortable doing. However, you will eventually have to shift your training to a slightly higher gear to continue to make progress and lose fat.

This chapter is going to give you a full training plan based on the diet you choose to follow and also how this will affect your performance and goals.

SKD Training Plans

On the SKD you'll be following a pretty straightforward nutrition scheme. As long as you keep your carbs low and fat high, you'll be in ketosis and make progress. Given the abrupt switch though its probably a good idea to take things slow and ease into training, even if you're someone who's used to training a lot. Let's break it down on a weekly basis and look at what you can expect and how you can tailor your training accordingly.

Week 1

Week 1 begins with you adopting the keto diet. Ideally, you should do this over a weekend or two consecutive non-training days. You should have your macros figured out in advance and have everything ready to go. We'll go over your meal plan later so don't fret if you're worried about planning your meals.

The first week is usually characterized by the dreaded keto fog. You will feel lethargic and sluggish and you won't be able to sleep very well. The first week is also where you will lose a lot of weight. However, this is just excess water being drained since you're restricting carbs.

In light of this, you should ensure your water intake is high since you will be shedding a lot of it and your body hasn't fully adjusted to using less water than is usually available. Also, it's a good idea to go slow in training this week. You should be keenly aware of getting exhausted and overtraining and not exceed these limits.

Don't be discouraged by the drop in training performance, you'll make it back within a week's time. While you need to be aware of lethargy and a general lack of energy, resist the temptation to skip training altogether. Training forces your body even more to burn fat instead of glucose and will bring you into ketosis faster. The faster you enter ketosis, the quicker you'll be rid of the mental fog.

This doesn't mean you train like a maniac. Go easy and find a good balance. This is also the first time you'll be maintaining a caloric deficit. The keto diet takes some adjusting to mentally at first because you'll be eating a far lesser quantity of food than you're accustomed to, even if you're eating the same number of calories. Remember, a gram of fat releases 9kcal of energy as opposed to 4 kcal per gram for carbs.

Therefore, it's logical that you'll need to eat lesser fat to gain the same amount of energy as carbs. Your meal sizes will shrink and you'll probably second guess yourself because of this. Always monitor your mood. If you're feeling lethargic, this is normal. If you feel short tempered and stressed out and find yourself irritated constantly, you've made a mistake calculating your macros and need to eat more food.

For those of you who will be training for the first time, pick an activity you've always wanted to do and start doing it. Running, swimming, playing a sport, cycling, whatever it is, just start moving and breaking a sweat. If you'll be hitting the gym, stick to the treadmills, ellipticals and stationary bikes for now and perform these exercises for 45 minutes at a comfortable speed. The key is to ease yourself into this new regime and not shock yourself into it.

You will feel sore after your workout and this is good. This is how your body becomes stronger and fitter. During the first week, it's best if you train on alternate days for 3 or 4 days. Pick any time of the day that is convenient for you and always eat a meal within an hour of finishing training.

Week 2

You should be back to normal by this time or towards the end of the previous week. If you're still having problems, try working out fasted for a day to see if your body adjusts. If you're still having issues there are two possible issues. Either you've miscalculated your macros and are eating far too less or your body is simply refusing to adjust due to some condition you are not aware of. If its the latter case, consult your doctor immediately and act as they advise.

If you're back to normal levels, this is great news! You can continue training the way you have been, prior to adopting the diet. If you were not training before, continue what you were doing on week 1. If you feel up to it, try increasing the length of your workout or increase the number of days while keeping the same workout length.

This week is all about feeling good and observing how you're adapting to your new diet. So keep working near your limit while simultaneously discovering how much you can push against it.

As a reminder, you'll be performing aerobic cardio activities this week as well. It's still too soon to transition to weight training.

Week 3

This is the week where you will first begin to push your limits and really start testing yourself. This doesn't have to be strenuous, mind you. If you find yourself becoming irritable or stressed out, remember, this means you're eating too less and have miscalculated your macros. So always be on the lookout for this.

By this point, you will have noticed that you feel hungry most of the time. This is not a rabid hunger but your stomach will feel lighter than usual and your brain will keep telling you that you can accommodate a little more food in there. This is happening because you're in a caloric deficit. If you've never experienced this before, it will be a weird sensation for you to not eat when you're hungry.

Again, this is worth repeating: monitor your mood constantly. If you constantly feel stressed out and irritable or burned out, you're eating too less. If this is the case eat more. Your hunger should not be more than a mild one. If you had to put words to it it would probably be "I could eat more but I can manage this".

From a training perspective, this week is when you will need to start lifting weights. Ideally, you will begin a strength training program of your choice. When picking a program, remember the guidelines set out in the previous chapter and pick something that is simple and easy to follow and incorporates progressive overload principles. You will be starting light, with an empty bar, so take it easy and continue as you previously were with your aerobic exercise.

Also, limit your workouts to 4 days per week. Recovery is where the most progress is made NOT during workouts. Most beginners fail to recognize this and workout to insane schedules. Rest and recovery are as essential as working out. Rest when you're supposed to and workout when you should. Discipline is not just performing an action when you need to but also involves doing nothing when the time is called for it.

Week 4

You're well into ketosis by now and you should be seeing its effect on the weighing scale. If you aren't seeing any progress, don't worry. You're probably not maintaining enough of a deficit. So reduce your meal portions a bit and see how that works. On the other hand, if you find you've gained weight, you're obviously eating too much to reduce your portions and monitor how that goes.

As far as workouts go, you should be well established into a schedule by now. Your strength training will be to approach challenging levels by the end of this week and you will begin to feel exhausted by your workouts. This is a good time to reduce your aerobic exercises and limit them to perhaps 10-15 minutes at the most after your workout.

You might be bummed out by this if you really love cycling or running but this will pay dividends in the long run so stick to the method. Your increased strength will give you more energy to perform better at those activities.

Week 5

This is where your training becomes very challenging and most people will start stalling on their weights at this point. This represents literally the first time your body has hit its limits and is now pushing past them so its a time to celebrate!

You should have a handle on your diet by now in terms of eyeballing how much you need to eat to maintain your macros and you should have a rough idea of whether you've eaten the correct amount by observing your hunger pangs, the degree of them that is.

If you feel up to it, try alternating between HIIT and steady state cardio at the end of your workouts. If HIIT is too strenuous, leave it be. Remember, your HIIT workout should last a maximum of 10 minutes.

Week 6

By this point, you should have lost at least 4 pounds of fat and your body weight should reflect this. If you're examining yourself in the mirror, you should see changes in the areas where you usually *don't* accumulate fat. These areas are usually the ones which tone up first.

Given the strength training you're doing, you should be seeing some physical changes from that as well. If you're squatting correctly, you will notice your legs becoming thicker and stronger. Your upper back will also have some definition by now and the deadlifts will have affected your posterior quite a bit by now.

At this point, it is crucial to continue observing your body and most importantly, identify the differences between being sore and an injury. Sometimes, in the excitement of all these changes, you will push a little too hard and tweak something. When you're sore, you will find it hard to move the muscle and there will be some pain but if you perform the movement that produced the soreness, you'll find that it goes away.

With an injury, the pain is constant and performing the movement only makes it worse. Those of you performing the bench press for the first time will feel this soreness in your chest. Don't mistake this for an injury. If you continue to perform the movement, it'll go away.

Week 7

By this point, you should have lost at least 5 pounds if you've done things correctly. If not, tweak your macros and observe what is helping and what is hindering and act accordingly.

If you've been experimenting with HIIT, you should be finding it a bit easier by now. Continue to push the limits by testing the work and rest interval timings. If you find HIIT a challenge but not an overwhelming one, you can drop steady state cardio at this point. This has the added benefit of reducing your overall workout time as well.

Week 9

Yes, we've skipped a week since by this point things should be in control for you. Hopefully, you've reached a stage where you're stalling for a second time in your strength training.

This is also the point where you will observe that you're losing lesser weight at a slower rate than previously. This is a very good sign if it happens because it means you've reached a stage where the most stubborn fat is clinging onto you. Once this fat leaves, there's not much more left!

The reason this happens is that you've lost enough weight to throw off your macros and your deficit. You see, since you're at a lower weight, your BMR is at a lower level and your deficit is lower. So simply recalculate your ratios and off you go!

This is how you handle the dreaded fat loss plateau which you may have read about. Most people make the mistake of increasing their activity level but remember what we learned earlier. Fat loss is almost entirely dependent on your diet, not your workout routine.

What has also happened is that your body has become much more efficient at producing fuel for itself so it is using whatever food you provide a lot more efficiently. The more efficient it becomes, the more it does with less. This does not mean you can indiscriminately reduce your food intake, of course.

Week 10

This is the point where all those around you will start noticing changes in you since they've become obvious by now. You'll need to start replacing your wardrobe soon!

Jokes apart, you simply need to stay the course at this point and just keep doing what you're doing.

Week 12

We're nearing the 3-month mark now and its time to take stock of your situation. You've probably lost around 10 pounds of fat by now. You're maintaining a healthy caloric deficit with your diet. You should be around the intermediate level with your strength training.

At this point, with regards to strength training, a beginner level routine will not help you much and you face a choice to either start an intermediate routine or maintain your levels and instead add other activities you enjoy. So if you've had to give up some cycling or swimming to train in the gym more, this is the time you pick that back up.

You reduce your strength training in the gym to 3 days and lift the same weight as close to your stalling points as possible and indulge in the other activities. You will find a marked improvement in those given the changes you've made.

Alternatively, you can continue on an intermediate program and add some split training routines. If you do this you will have to increase the number of days you train. Also, remember to keep doing your HIIT or steady state cardio, whichever it is you find useful.

Given that your body has been on a deficit for three months, its time to allow it to recover a bit. You see, being on a deficit for longer than this not healthy. So recalculate your macros and start eating at maintenance levels and always keep a track of your body weight. If you find yourself putting on weight, you're eating too much. If you're losing weight, you're eating too less. Your weight should stay the same more or less within a pound. You need to eat at maintenance for a couple of months and then get back onto a deficit to further cut fat if you need to.

Alternatively, if you're happy with the way you look, you can try bulking up via the HPKD or TKD and increase your muscle mass.

Either way, congratulations! You've discovered how simple weight loss and fat loss really is !

Chapter 7: HPKD Training Plan

We've looked at the aims of the HPKD previously and how, if your objective is to increase the amount of muscle, that is to bulk up, the HPKD is the best diet for you to follow. With this diet you will be running a caloric surplus, that is you will be eating more than your maintenance level requires.

This caloric excess does not mean you have a free license to eat any old junk. You still need to follow the basic of good nutrition and watch what you eat. The HPKD is more fun to follow than the SKD though due to this reason.

We'll now take a look at your training plan on a weekly basis. There are some assumptions which have been made here. One is that if you're looking to bulk up, you've already had some experience training and know your way around a gym. While your experience doesn't have to be extensive, you can start strength training immediately and don't need to perform aerobic cardio to increase your base strength.

If this is not the case, the SKD is recommended for you since you probably don't have the muscle to begin with and will probably end up with middling results by following this diet routine.

So having made that clear, let's dive in!

HPKD Training Plans

Since the HPKD calls for maintaining an excess of calories, you won't find this very taxing mentally. However, you will need to hit the gym hard and regularly because those excess calories, if not burned to fuel muscles, will turn into fat, defeating the purpose of following the diet in the first place.

Week 1

Just like with the SKD, the best way to begin the HPKD is by adopting it over a weekend or over two non-training days to give yourself ample time to adjust to the new diet regime. Prior to beginning its best to have all your supplements sorted out, especially fiber supplements since the combination of higher protein and low carbs pretty much remove all fiber from your diet.

Your workouts should not be fasted under any circumstances. Since the aim of this diet is to aid in muscle gain, working out fasted will inhibit muscle growth. While there's no set time for you to workout, aim to do so on a full stomach.

Your workout themselves should be a combination of strength training, depending on your strength level this can be beginner or intermediate level programs, and isolation exercises. A word of caution though: if you're not yet at an intermediate level of strength then sticking to beginner strength program and building your strength up to intermediate standards is the best way forward.

Timing your cardio sessions is of great importance if you're looking to build muscle. To this effect, it's best to perform cardio prior to your workouts for around 10-15 minutes. Doing so after your workouts will only cause greater stress to be placed on your muscles and you will risk muscle loss, even if you're running a caloric surplus.

The only program to absolutely avoid is HIIT. You will be training at a pretty high-intensity level to begin with so HIIT would just be overkill and your gains will just take longer to be realized.

Week 2

You should be fully adjusted to your new diet by now. If the keto fog still persists, take the same steps as advised while doing the SKD, that is, figure out if you've calculated your macros correctly and if so, then consult your doctor about the efficacy of the diet.

If you are properly adjusted then as far as your workout goes, its best to continue your current program and to keep progressively increasing the weight. Remember to finish your cardio pre-workout and do not do so post workout since this will limit your gains.

Week 4

This is an important week in terms of taking stock of where your progress is at in terms of target weight and workout performance. This week marks a month since you started the diet and the first thing to measure is your weight.

Remember that by maintaining a caloric excess, you're targeting a gain of 1 pound per week. Now not all of this will be muscle but by eating healthy and closely following workout principles, you will minimize fat gain and maximize your muscle gains. So the first thing to see is whether you've been putting on weight as per expected guidelines.

If you find yourself below your projected weight at this point, you ought to increase the calories you're eating by around 250 kcal. If you're overweight, reduce your consumption by 250 kcal. Next, you need to determine whether this increased weight is fat or muscle predominantly.

You could do a body composition test which a lot of clinics offer and get it done scientifically. If this seems like overkill to you, an easy way to determine this is to look at your workouts. Are you lifting heavier weight than when you began? How much heavier? Have you stalled recently? Ideally, you wouldn't have stalled up until now and your lifting weight at a far higher level than when you began.

This is, perhaps, a more artistic method of determining fat vs muscle so don't be alarmed or overreact to whatever you find. It's still too early to determine all this and this is merely a checkpoint to make sure you're on track.

We'll cover more on the topic of tracking and measurement in a later chapter so you will understand how to measure and more importantly what and when to measure.

Week 6

This week is when you'll begin stalling on your lifts and you will begin to find cardio a lot tougher to perform. If you find your stress levels increasing too much, to the extent that you're dreading your workouts, reduce your cardio sessions to once or twice a week.

Performing strength exercises at high intensity will build your anaerobic capacity so your cardio system will get a good workout. The idea is to maximize muscle gains which in turn will burn food more efficiently and reduce your fat gains. So always keep this objective in mind.

As for your lifts, a good idea to stimulate growth is to perform a single, heavy rep at the end of your sets. So if you're squatting 5X5, add a 6th set of 1 rep at the end with a weight that you think is too heavy, within a reasonable distance of where you're actually lifting right now. For example, if you're squatting 250 pounds and are close to stalling out, load 275 pounds on the bar. It's not necessary for you to actually squat this weight (if you think you can with the help of a spotter, do so) but at the very least balance it for a few seconds.

What this does is it gets your body and mind used to the idea that it can carry this much weight. A lot of weight lifting is mental and you'll be surprised at how much smoother your gains become by incorporating this technique.

Your diet should be on autopilot by now and you should be at the point where you can eyeball your portions and estimate whether it's too much or too less. It is essential for you to get adequate sleep and rest. Remember, muscle is gained and fat is burned when you rest, not when you workout.

Week 10

You will be approaching your second level of stalling on weights by this point. If you're not there yet, don't worry, you'll soon arrive. Once you stall and reload towards the weight again (every strength training program will explain what this is and how to do it. This is a diet book and hence, this process is beyond our scope), you will need to start planning our how you wish to take your training forward.

You could adopt an intermediate training program or, like in the SKD, you could maintain the weight levels and start engaging in other activities like cycling, running, sports etc. Either way, make sure you recalculate your macro levels and make sure you eat at maintenance.

You'll find your levels have changed and you will also need to factor in a higher activity level so do keep that in mind. Performing a full body composition test is a good idea at this point to determine how many pounds of muscle versus fat you have gained.

It bears mentioning at this point that those of you who have bulked on a carb-heavy diet will find that amount of muscle you have gained will be lesser than what you've observed previously. So why adopt the HPKD to bulk you might ask? This is a good question and it ultimately comes down to how well you think you can shed the fat you've gained during bulking.

If you find shedding the fat easy, then perhaps a carb heavy diet will be better suited for your bulk. However, if you have always struggled to shed the extra fat and during cutting, have always ended up losing muscle and ending up with a skinny fat look, then the HPKD will give you better results during the bulk since you'll be far more used to eating fat (as opposed to excess carbs) and your body will be completely adjusted to burning fat for fuel instead of having to re-adjust again.

If you're already at an advanced level and want to achieve the double advantage of losing fat and building muscle at the same time, then you need to get on the CKD or TKD. The CKD can be adopted by beginners as well who are having trouble getting adjusted to the high-fat requirements of the keto diet. We'll look at this next.

Chapter 8: CKD and TKD Training Plans

As we've seen previously, the CKD and TKD involve fueling yourself with carbs with an aim to replenish your glycogen stores to fuel your workouts or in the case o the CKD, to gently immerse yourself into the keto diet with an aim of going fully onto the SKD within a period of time.

Both objectives have very different goals and indeed, a very different audience. With this view, we will be looking at training plans for beginners, new to the keto diet, on the CKD and the training for more experienced people who can use either the CKD or TKD.

We'll first look at the beginners on the CKD

Beginners' CKD Training Plan

If you're new to the keto diet and are having troubles for whatever reason in adapting to the lesser carbs required or if you feel a gentler introduction to the keto diet would serve you better, then following the CKD for a period of 2-3 weeks is ideal.

As a refresher, the CKD calls for you to load on carbs on 2 days out of 7 and follow the SKD on the remaining 5. Since you're a beginner, you'll be maintaining a caloric deficit, no matter what you're eating so do keep that in mind.

Week 1

You will need to calculate two sets of macros for the CKD, one for the carbs heavy days and one for the SKD days. Remember, carb loading doesn't mean you get to binge on whatever you want. The CKD plan doesn't allow you to have any cheat days so you will be maintaining a deficit on all 7 days (We'll talk about cheat days more in the next few chapters).

Ideally, you should have your carb days coincide with your final workout day for the week and the day right after that. Another good option is to have the first carb day coincide with the rest day prior to the final workout of the week and the 2nd carb day be the day of the final workout itself. This way, you're properly fueled for the workout and can begin to prepare to enter ketosis soon after.

Given the 2 days you'll be eating carbs, you should not have much of a keto fog effect going on. If you do still experience it, consult your doctor. Remember to monitor your stress and mood levels and see if you've calculated your macros correctly and are eating right.

For your workouts, if you've never exercised before, begin with steady state aerobic cardio activities for this week and the next. If you are more experienced than a rank beginner, you may begin strength training with an empty bar and start working your way up.

Week 2

The second week of the CKD is pretty much the same as the previous one. You will continue to follow the diet guidelines and keep monitoring your mood and stress levels in case you're eating less.

If you were only performing cardio the previous week, continue to do so this week as well. You can try to increase the length of your workout for up to an hour this week. Don't worry if you can't go that long, the aim is to progressively increase your work levels.

You will be working out at least 4 days a week this week if you're not strength training.

Week 3

This will be your final week eating carbs before switching fully over to the SKD. If you feel comfortable doing so earlier than this feel free to do so. This week the only major change you will be making is, you will be eating carbs only one day of the week. This will be the day of your final workout of the week.

Again, this is not an excuse to binge or think that this is a final meal of sorts and lose self-control. Monitor yourself the days after this carb meal and see how you're taking it and adjusting to the SKD full time.

If you're finding some levels of fog occurring, this is normal and will probably persist for a week, albeit its occurrence is pretty rare. If this fog lasts for a longer time than that, the keto diet is probably not for you and you should consult a doctor to get your symptoms checked out.

For those who are able to adjust successfully, which is usually the majority of people, you can start following the SKD from week 3 onwards in the previous chapter and also keep increasing your workout activities as per the guidelines explained in that chapter.

TKD/CKD Training Plan

For more experienced people, that is those who are used to working out and have dieted in one form or another in the past, the TKD is a great option as opposed to an SKD due to the dual benefit of cutting fat and building muscle.

While you can adopt the CKD as well, your rate of fat loss will be low with this. The only exception is if you're a very experienced trainer, in which case you will hardly need a book to tell you what to do.

In the below sections, we'll address both options, the CKD and TKD, equally so you can get a better idea of which option might work for you best. Also, to make it abundantly clear, you will be eating at maintenance on this regime.

Week 1

If you choose to follow the TKD, this week will be more challenging than on the CKD. Remember to consume only up to 30 g carbs prior to your workout and not more. The idea is to have the carbs fuel your workout and then post workout, have your body hasten back into ketosis as soon as possible.

The type of workout you choose to follow will dictate the amount of carbs you choose to consume pre-workout. A good idea is to track the number of calories you regularly burn as part of a typical workout and aim to eat enough carbs to cover 3/4ths of that.

If you're on the CKD, remember to consume lesser carbs on the second day than the first in order to push yourself into ketosis sooner. Generally, the CKD is a less efficient way of achieving the dual goal of increased muscle and lower fat so it is advisable to switch to the TKD is convenient. You will still hit your goals if done properly but it will just take longer.

Week 3

Week 3 is a good point at which you can begin HIIT. As a rule, perform your cardio whenever you feel comfortable doing so and whichever gives you the best performance. Since you're in maintenance, it is not advisable to skip cardio since you might end up gaining some fat. As a rule of thumb, do steady state cardio prior to your workout and HIIT after your workout.

For those on CKD, you will need to be performing HIIT fasted the day after your second carb day. You can choose to do this in the morning and workout in the evening or combine the two into one morning workout. No approach is superior to another, so go with whatever works best for you.

This is also the point where, should you choose, you can switch over to the TKD. A pertinent question to consider here is are you better off working out fasted or not? The answer, again, is do whatever you can sustain for the longest. A fasted workout is mentally more taxing and while you can will your way through a few days or even weeks, eventually, it catches up to you. Consistency is what brings results so do whatever you can maintain the longest for.

Week 6

You have probably stalled a couple times on your lifts by now and must be approaching your strength limits. Generally, it is not advisable at this point to change your activities. Instead, adopt an intermediate level strength program and follow that for more gains.

This applies to both CKD and TKD options. As always keep tracking your weight and if you're seeing any significant weight gain or loss, adjust your macros accordingly.

Week 8

At this point, you should be seeing physical changes in the mirror. Keep doing what you're doing. To be perfectly honest, at an intermediate level, you will not see huge changes like those at a beginner's stage. It will be boring and that's perfectly OK.

Week 12

At this point, you need to take stock of your gains and your goals. If need be, this is where you can choose to maintain your strength level and branch out into different activities like sports or cycling, running and other activities you usually enjoy. As always make sure to take your activity level into consideration when calculating your energy needs.

This concludes our look at the training plan and schedules with respect to the SKD, HPKD, TKD, and CKD. As you may have noticed, there are lesser things to worry about as you make progress largely because a lot of it becomes second nature to you. This is why persistence pays off and making progress will become second nature to you.

You will have noticed there are a quite a few things to track and this might be intimidating for you if you're just starting out. With this in mind, in the next chapter, we will take a look at everything to do with tracking and recording progress.

Chapter 9: Tracking

You will not make progress in anything that you do not track. When starting out, tracking will feel tedious because you've probably never bothered to do so. This chapter will give you everything you need to know about not just what to track, but also how and when to track them.

Without further ado, let's jump right in and look at the things you need to track from a diet perspective.

Diet Tracking

There are a few things you have to track when following your chosen keto diet. Some of them are obvious and some are not. The good news is from a diet perspective there really isn't all that much to do and most of it becomes repetitive after a couple weeks.

In fact, you'll probably be able to eyeball all of these without the need for any measuring because you'll get adjusted to it.

Ingredient Portions

This is the major thing you need to track as part of any diet, not just keto. Your best investment with this view will be a food weighing scale. This way you will be able to measure your portions in grams or pounds.

Another good idea is to purchase measuring cups for fluids. Given the demands of the diet, you will be eating more cream and fatty oils so measuring these out is essential. Remember, you get a lot more energy from a gram of fat than carbs and protein so at first, you will not be able to eyeball how much you think you need.

Calorie Count

Using any free calorie tracker (like FitDay for example) is absolutely necessary. Not only do these software make it easy for you to track your calories but they also help enforce discipline by forcing you to engage in your progress.

This really should be a no-brainer but you'd be surprised at the number of people who neglect this and squander all progress. Another rookie mistake that people make is to think that they need to enter food into this software every single day.

The key to making any diet regime work is to make it as repeatable and simple as possible. This means if you're comfortable with entering your food into this every time you eat, then great. If you find this tedious and irritating, then you need to set up your process to be as repeatable as possible. We'll look at this in greater detail in the next chapter but one way of doing this is to reduce the number of raw ingredients from which you will cook your meals to a small number.

This way you know the calorie counts of all the ingredients and cooking your meals simply becomes a case of mixing and matching them. Alternatively, you could simply eat the same thing every day for a while and when you get bored of it, change it up with a new set of ingredients and calculate your macros for the new foods.

Mental State

While this is a bit nebulous to track, in that there are no numbers involved, it is just as important to track. Your levels of stress and moods are key indicators in helping you figure out whether you're headed in the right direction or not. If your caloric deficit is too high, this will always manifest as irritability and stress or the feeling of being burned out.

Ketone Levels

Tracking your ketone levels is also a good idea since this will let you know how your body reacts specifically to certain types of food. Everyone is built differently and determining the number of carbs that cause you to exit ketosis will make your life a whole lot easier. Once you've determined this level, set this as your carb level in your macro calculation and add food as appropriate.

The best way of tracking your ketones is via a weekly average method. You could choose any one of the measuring techniques detailed previously and throughout the week consume the number of carbs you've set for yourself as per your macro calculation. If you find you're not able to maintain ketosis then you will need to decrease the carbs consumed.

On the other hand, if you're able to maintain ketosis, you could choose to increase your carb intake slightly, by say 10g per day, and look at the cumulative effect. This way, you can test your carb limit for ketosis and design your diet accordingly. It is not necessary for you to be at your carb limit but consuming a higher number of carbs could help you adjust to the keto diet better.

Workout Tracking

There are a number of things you should be tracking when it comes to your workouts. Some of these are not strictly workout related but are important nonetheless.

Weight

Throughout the previous chapters, we've seen how tracking your weight is essential in determining your progress. To this effect, a weighing scale is a must buy along with the previously mentioned food weighing scale.

Always weigh yourself at the same time every day. So if you decide to weigh yourself right after waking up, on an empty stomach, always weight yourself at this time for as long as you're on the diet. You will find that your weight, on a day to day basis, will fluctuate. A lot of this has to do with water weight and other miscellaneous items that cause water retention or excretion.

Therefore, when you compare your weights across weeks, always compare the average weight NOT the day to day weight numbers. If you find that your average weight per week is reducing at a rate of 1 pound per week, this is a good sign. Don't pay much heed to the daily numbers, remember it is the average that counts.

Waist Size

You can track your other physical measurements, like chest/bust, biceps, neck and so on but tracking your waist size is extremely important. More than anything else, this indicates your level of fat loss.

Just like with your weight, measure this at the same time every day and pay attention to the weekly average number.

Exercise Weight

When you head to the gym, you need to carry a log book with you. This log will have the exercises you intend on performing that session, the sets and reps and the weight you intend to lift for that exercise. If you're performing cardio, it needs to record the intended session length.

Once you actually perform the exercises, you check off each set and rep and log whether you were able to complete that task or not. This logging is extremely important in any strength training program since you'll be increasing the weight on a regular basis.

Calories Burned

While this number is not strictly necessary, if you use a Fitbit or any other activity tracker, it is helpful to use them to track your heart rate and calories burned during your workouts.

This, in turn, will help you determine whether your BMR numbers, which you estimate your diet macros off of, are accurate or not.

These are the important metric that you should be tracking at a bare minimum. Remember to keep reviewing these on a weekly basis to confirm whether you are on track or not. Any counter indications mean you need to go back and recalculate your macros and adjust your portions.

Next, we will look at the various aspects of meal prep and how you can do this easily.

Chapter 10: Keto Meal Prep

Now that you understand how to incorporate exercise plans into your lifestyle along with tracking your stats, all that remains to be looked at is meal prep. This is an area most people let themselves down in due to inconsistency and due to generally overlooking this.

When sitting down to figure out your meals, you'll probably go online and search for recipes and pick the ones that sound the most enticing. While there's nothing wrong with this approach, what most people ignore are the ramifications for their shopping list and the demands on time most of these diverse recipes call for.

With this in mind, let's now look at how to go about prepping your meals so that you don't have to sacrifice on taste and use your time in the most efficient manner possible.

Keto Staples

The success or failure of any diet regime depends on how consistently you can enforce it. Following a diet is not about restricting yourself or saying "I can't eat this". Instead, it is looking at all the things you CAN do and reducing that list of things to the most repeatable and easy ones for you to follow.

You can look at various cookbooks and online recipes and come up with any number of recipes, all of which will be undoubtedly delicious. However, if these recipes require you to cook each and every one of them, every single time, you probably are not spending your time wisely.

If you have the time and inclination to cook then, of course, there's no problem. However, for most of us, work and other demands take up a significant amount of time. The best course of action is to reduce the diet to a few staples and mix these with a few rotating cast members, so to speak. The staples vegans need to stock up on are pretty self-explanatory since the majority of these are plant sourced. Generally speaking, there isn't anything special vegans need to do beyond prepare alternate protein sources.

This way your meal prep is reduced to a few minutes at the most and will involve either reheating or putting together your meal. So what are some of these staples?

Salad Greens

Salads are simple and straightforward to prepare. Chop up your favorite veggies and toss them into a bowl and let them mix together. It's always a good idea to mix a big batch of salad greens together and store it in your fridge for further use. Salads by themselves are not very calorie dense and therefore, you need not worry about getting your portion size exactly right.

They're relatively easy to spice up as well! Toss in some onions or jalapenos to spice it up. Alternatively, you could put together a batch of homemade pico de gallo (tomatoes, onions, peppers, cilantro) and divide it into meal portions.

Baked Chicken Breast or Thighs

Chicken is generally viewed as the most boring of meats and chicken breast is the least exciting bit of the bird. While all this is true, it is also, like most boring things, one of the healthiest proteins you can consume. You don't need to stand at the stove every single time to cook this. Simply bake a batch of them and reheat it for your meals portion-wise.

Baking, you will find, is one of the best ways to reduce your time in the kitchen and still have tasty meals ready to go. You could bake pretty much anything, including your vegetables or other meat. It is recommended to limit your red meat intake due to the previously mentioned saturated fat content in them. Once a week is perfectly fine though. If you're younger, say below the age of 25, then you can increase this pretty safely.

Chicken is an especially good option since it doesn't tend to lose its flavor when reheated, unlike other meat and fish. Turkey, for example, will often dry out easily when reheating and you might as well eat leather than eat reheated steak. Pairing your chicken breast with salads is an easy meal option.

Chicken thighs contain a higher amount of saturated fat and are tastier than chicken breast cuts. It's perfectly fine to consume chicken thighs as long as you minimize your consumption of them. In other words, instead of eating them every day, consume them as much as you would red meat.

Keto Snacks

The snacks are perhaps the best bit about the keto diet. Given the abundance of fat the diet calls for, a whole world of possibilities opens up. You could go wild with bacon wrapped snacks and other exotic options but for consistency's sake, and if you don't have too much time to cook and prep your meals, a few staples will serve you well.

Dark chocolate and peanut butter along with some fatty nuts and dry fruits will fill you up more often than not. You can choose to combine these ingredients in any way possible. This is especially satisfying if you happen to have a sweet tooth. A dessert of peanut butter mixed with dark chocolate topped with whipped cream can rival anything a fancy restaurant has to offer.

Keto Bread and Tortillas

One of the things most people struggle to get used to is the lack of grains in the keto diet. Most of us are used to eating rice or wheat in some form or another and find it difficult to feel full on just a salad.

With this in mind, it's a great idea to whip up a batch of keto bread or tortillas. These are made with coconut flour and you can find the recipes for the online quite easily. Store these away and you can now make pretty much anything from quesadillas to sandwiches to even pancakes for breakfast!

For those who prefer rice, whipping up a batch of keto rice, that is dehydrated cauliflower rice, is a good option. You should be careful with the portion sizes though since it could put you over your carb limits pretty easily.

The recipes for all of these are easily available if you search online or in any good ketogenic recipe books.

Eggs

When in doubt, have some eggs. Don't feel like cooking anything? Have some eggs. Meal feels a bit light? Feeling hungrier than usual? Have some eggs.

Eggs are an excellent source of fat and protein. Make sure you eat the yolk along with the whites. While it is true that the yolk will have a negative effect on your cholesterol levels, with proper exercise, as you will be doing, this risk is minimized so eat the whole egg.

Cheese

The previous section on eggs could be repeated word for word when it comes to cheese. A word of caution though: You should pay attention to what sort of cheese you are consuming. These days, given the proliferation of processed food, you will find a lot of cheeses made from vegetable oil and not from milk. Needless to stay, do not consume these.

Stick to a few base kinds of cheese like parmesan, ricotta, cheddar, and mozzarella. These are high in protein and are tasty to boot. You can also try cream cheese but most of these are highly processed so minimize your intake of these. Cottage cheese or farmer's cheese are also great options along with feta, halloumi and other Mediterranean and Levantine cheeses. Just make sure these are deli cheeses and not your garden variety supermarket counter cheese.

A word on processing: We've looked at this before but it bears repeating. All cheese is "processed". There is, however, a big difference between chemical processing and the processing that occurs as a natural part of the fermenting process. When you read about processing it refers to the chemical and other processing that doesn't make sense. For example, who ever heard of cheese coming from vegetables? So why would you consume cheese made from vegetable fat?

Sardines or Tuna

Tuna is an old favorite of bodybuilders everywhere. It also happens to taste disgustingly bad. With this in mind, you could switch to sardines or mackerel. Sardines are a great, cheap and easy option to cook and add to your salads. You could also add anchovies or other dried fish.

Always keep a can of tuna or sardines handy in case you run out of food or feel too tired to put together a full meal.

In addition to the above you also want to stock up your kitchen with the foods below:

- Nuts and seeds
- Nut butters
- Herbs
    - Thyme

    - Oregano
    - Garlic powder
    - Parsley
    - Dill
    - Salt and pepper
- Coconut flour
- Coconut Cream
- Healthy oils like
    - Olive Oil (refer to earlier sections regarding pomace versus extra virgin)
    - Coconut oil
    - Sesame oil
- Baking powder
- Mayonnaise

Foods to Minimize

The foods below are fully allowed on the keto diet but most people tend to take this as a free license to binge on these. Watch your portions when consuming these foods and minimize them as much as possible.

Heavy Cream

It's the easiest source of fat you can find and it's equally easy to dunk everything into a pot of cream. Go easy on this because the cream is the last thing you want to overeat.

Bacon

Everybody's favorite food is fully allowed on the keto diet. Searching recipes online will yield you a large majority of bacon-based recipes and most people forget to limit their intake of it. Bacon is full of saturated fat so you should minimize your intake of it, even if a daily dose of bacon falls within your macros.

Artificial Sweetener

Sugar is completely out on the keto diet so most people, especially those who drink a lot of coffee or tea, feel compelled to add artificial sweeteners to their drink. Again, these are not naturally occurring foods so you should be very careful in limiting your intake of these. Stevia and the like are processed foods so, in the short term, a little bitterness in your coffee will pay dividends over the long run.

Red Meat

While delicious, red meat has a high amount of saturated fat and you should be minimizing this. While some amount of saturated fat is good for us, an excess is clearly bad. The answer, therefore, as we say in the chapter on nutrition basics, is to minimize red meat and not cut it out completely. Stick to the leaner cuts of meat and consume this once or twice a week and you'll be fine.

Diet Design

We've already looked at the major points of designing a diet. This involves determining your activity levels and then based on your BMR, you need to calculate your macros at a deficit, maintenance or an excess depending on your goals.

A good idea when designing a diet is to add in cheat meals once a week. This cheat meal is not a license to binge but it is a day when you can relax your calorie consumption limit and can maybe go over your carb limit just a bit. Moderation is the key to this and is a point most people forget.

Another important point to keep in mind is that all calorie counts you see on software and your BMR rates etc are all estimates. They are not accurate down to the final calorie. This is why it is essential for you to constantly monitor your weight on a weekly basis. If you've observed that your mean weight has been increasing, its not a reason to panic or to beat yourself up. Instead, simply cut your calorie consumption by 250 kcal and track from there on out. Similarly, if you're losing too much weight, that is greater than 1 pound per week, you're eating too less and increase your intake by 250 kcal.

So for example, if you are really craving a pizza, instead of eating a full medium sized pie, have just a slice. Take your time to really savor it. Remember, if your diet feels overly restrictive and is causing you a lot of stress to keep up with, it's probably not for you. The best diet is one that you can follow.

There will always be some restrictive feeling whenever you begin a new diet or are disciplining yourself. You should not confuse this feeling with one of stress. If even after a month of following a new diet regimen, you find yourself dreading meal time or are spending an inordinate amount of time thinking and worrying about what you're eating, then it's probably an indication that this diet is not for you.

If you're on the CKD, a cheat meal really isn't necessary since the diet itself is a compromise so do keep that in mind.

Above all else, remember the first principle of dieting: Always design something that is as repeatable as possible. This is why we've looked at staples and exercise regimes that are basic and can be implemented with the least amount of effort. Dieting and disciplining yourself is tough to begin with. You owe it to yourself to make this as smooth as possible.

Tools for Starting Meal Prep

In addition to the staple foods listed above, you will need the following kitchen equipment to get up and running:

- Skillet
- Quality Knife
- Slow cooker or crockpot
- Parchment paper
- Baking dishes
- Food processor
- Food weighing scale and other tracking equipment as listed in the previous chapter

Purchasing a quality cast iron skillet along with a good chef's knife will reduce your meal prep times and simply make your life a whole lot easier when it comes to preparing your meals. The skillet will come in handy when you need to quickly prepare some eggs or bacon. Generally speaking, to minimize your time spent in the kitchen (assuming this is what you want), baking and slow cooking are your best options. The best slow cooker would be an Instant Pot where you can simply throw everything in and let it work its magic.

Food processors will help you with preparing great tasting carb substitutes like caulifower rice and in addition to this, you can also whip up some great options like seed butters, smoothies etc.

Steps to Successful Prep

Prepping your meals successfully is a pretty straightforward task as evidenced by the list below:

1. Plan your meals a week in advance
2. Plan cooking schedule (either cooked in advance of scratch)
3. Shop
4. Cook

Step 1 is the most important of all. It is necessary when you're starting out to plan everything in advance since you'll be dealing with a lot of other adjustments when you adopt the keto diet.

Plan your breakfasts, lunches and dinners along with a staple few snacks like nuts and butters, you will consume. As mentioned previously, to make this easy, repeat as many meals as possible. When choosing recipes, you can go online and search for recipes which already have the macros listed in them and easily calculate your portions.

While this helps in the short term, over the longer term, it pays to reduce your ingredients for the week to a few staples and then decide on the recipes from there, based on how much you would like to eat them. Relying on someone else's calorie counts will only lead to laziness and that's the last thing you want.

Step 2 is where you will decide when to cook your meals. Cook your meals in the easiest and most repeatable manner possible. While cooking in advance is tempting, its not a good idea to make your meals more than 2 days in advance. Storing cooked meals in the fridge will reduce the taste and in the case of red meat or chicken, change the texture of the meat and make it less tasty.

While convenience is important, don't follow it at the cost of making things hard on yourself. While out shopping, that is step 3, make sure to purchase quantities for the entire week. You can easily calculate this from step 1. Alternatively, you could work backwards from the quantity you would like to consume and design recipes around it. For example, if you prefer consuming 100 grams of chicken thighs everyday, purchase 1kg of thighs and store it in your freezer.

Prepping your meals and cooking them will take some adjusting to, especially if you're used to consuming foods from the center aisles of your department store (which is where all the processed foods are). Taking it slow and methodically mapping out each and every step is the key to success with this.

Conclusion

The ketogenic diet is a wonderful way to lose fat or gain muscle or even to do both simultaneously. The diet's requirements are quite basic and easy to follow. Allied with the right exercise program, you will see guaranteed results.

Remember to always keep the basics of nutrition and exercise in mind as you go about implementing this in your life. A caloric deficit is necessary for you to lose weight and a caloric excess is for gaining weight. Always track how much you're eating and also track the various parameters we looked at in the chapter on tracking. It is the average numbers you want to pay attention to, not the day to day numbers which will fluctuate.

Depending on your goals you can choose to adopt the SKD, HPKD, CKD or TKD. While the TKD and HPKD are for slightly more experienced people, you can always adopt them after following the SKD or CKD. It is important to be aware of your goals right from the start, whether it is to lose fat or gain muscle or recompose the lean muscle mass versus fat your body. If you're not able to decide on what you need first, asking those around you or going with your gut feeling is usually the best option.

Keep your shelves stocked with some keto staples and you will make your life a lot easier when it comes to making meals, especially if you don't have the time or inclination to spend a lot of time in the kitchen. Prepare these in batches and them together and you'll have tasty and nutritious meals ready in no time.

Revisiting the first few chapters regarding the basics of nutrition and exercise will do you a world of good. Initially, it will seem like a lot but keep at it and you will reap the rewards!

Thank you very much, once again, for purchasing this book. If you feel you've learned something useful and if this book has helped you take a step towards your goals, please do leave a review, it is much appreciated!

Bibliography

Chapter 1

1: Nutrition. (2019). Retrieved from https://www.who.int/topics/nutrition/en/

2: Water: How much should you drink every day?. (2019). Retrieved from https://www.mayoclinic.org/healthy-lifestyle/nutrition-and-healthy-eating/in-depth/water/art-20044256

Chapter 2

1: Mandal, A. (2019). History of the Ketogenic Diet. Retrieved from https://www.news-medical.net/health/History-of-the-Ketogenic-Diet.aspx

2,3: Foster, G., Wyatt, H., Hill, J., McGuckin, B., Brill, C., & Mohammed, B. et al. (2003). A Randomized Trial of a Low-Carbohydrate Diet for Obesity. New England Journal Of Medicine, 348(21), 2082-2090. doi: 10.1056/nejmoa022207

4,5: Brehm, B., Seeley, R., Daniels, S., & D'Alessio, D. (2003). A Randomized Trial Comparing a Very Low Carbohydrate Diet and a Calorie-Restricted Low Fat Diet on Body Weight and Cardiovascular Risk Factors in Healthy Women. The Journal Of Clinical Endocrinology & Metabolism, 88(4), 1617-1623. doi: 10.1210/jc.2002-021480

6,7: Daly, M., Paisey, R., Paisey, R., Millward, B., Eccles, C., & Williams, K. et al. (2006). Short-term effects of severe dietary carbohydrate-restriction advice in Type 2 diabetes-a randomized controlled trial. Diabetic Medicine, 23(1), 15-20. doi: 10.1111/j.1464-5491.2005.01760.x

8,9: Gasior, M., Rogawski, M. A., & Hartman, A. L. (2006). Neuroprotective and disease-modifying effects of the ketogenic diet. Behavioral Pharmacology, 17(5-6), 431-9.

10,11: Zhou, W., Mukherjee, P., Kiebish, M. A., Markis, W. T., Mantis, J. G., & Seyfried, T. N. (2007). The calorically restricted ketogenic diet, an effective alternative therapy for malignant brain cancer. Nutrition & Metabolism, 4, 5. doi:10.1186/1743-7075-4-5

12: Zhou, W., Mukherjee, P., Kiebish, M. A., Markis, W. T., Mantis, J. G., & Seyfried, T. N. (2007). The calorically restricted ketogenic diet, an effective alternative therapy for malignant brain cancer. Nutrition & Metabolism, 4, 5. doi:10.1186/1743-7075-4-5

13: Paoli, A., Grimaldi, K., Toniolo, L., Canato, M., Bianco, A., & Fratter, A. (2012). Nutrition and Acne: Therapeutic Potential of Ketogenic Diets. Skin Pharmacology And Physiology, 25(3), 111-117. doi: 10.1159/000336404

Chapter 3

1: Cronkleton, E., & Sullivan, D. (2019). What Happens If You Eat Too Much Protein?. Retrieved from https://www.healthline.com/health/too-much-protein#recommended-daily-protein

Chapter 5

1,2,3,4: McCall, P. (2019). 7 Things to Know About Excess Post-exercise Oxygen Consumption (EPOC). Retrieved from https://www.acefitness.org/education-and-resources/professional/expert-articles/5008/7-things-to-know-about-excess-post-exercise-oxygen-consumption-epoc

5,6: Veracity, D. (2019). Bone density sharply enhanced by weight training, even in the elderly. Retrieved from https://www.naturalnews.com/010528_bone_density_mineral.html

7: Long-term weight training may benefit Parkinson's disease patients. (2019). Retrieved from https://www.news-medical.net/news/20120217/Long-term-weight-training-may-benefit-Parkinsons-disease-patients.aspx

8: Schmitz, K., Ahmed, R., Troxel, A., Cheville, A., Smith, R., & Lewis-Grant, L. et al. (2009). Weight Lifting in Women with Breast-Cancer–Related Lymphedema. New England Journal Of Medicine, 361(7), 664-673. doi: 10.1056/nejmoa0810118

9: Häkkinen A, Häkkinen K, Hannonen P, et al. Strength training induced adaptations in neuromuscular function of premenopausal women with fibromyalgia: comparison with healthy women. Annals of the Rheumatic Diseases 2001;60:21-26.

10: De Backer, I., Van Breda, E., Vreugdenhil, A., Nijziel, M., Kester, A., & Schep, G. (2007). High-intensity strength training improves quality of life in cancer survivors. Acta Oncologica, 46(8), 1143-1151. doi: 10.1080/02841860701418838

www.ingramcontent.com/pod-product-compliance
Lightning Source LLC
Chambersburg PA
CBHW031154020426
42333CB00013B/660
9781950921119

Are you keen to lose weight and get in shape this year?

Have you decided that a combination of diet and exercise will help you achieve your goal?

The ketogenic diet could be the answer.

Many people want to lose weight. Unfortunately for most, they will try dieting for a week or two before they lose interest. This can often lead to cycle of dieting and binging, going back to old habits before deciding to try again.

Inside this book you will find all the inspiration you need to start your keto diet, complete with solid information and exercise routines that will give you great results with chapters on:

- **Keto diet**
- **Exercises for maximum fat burning**
- **Exercises for Toning**
- **Exercises for Building muscle**
- **Athletic training**
- **Keto Supplements**
- **Meal preparation for the keto diet**
- **And more…**

The keto diet offers a different option to most weight loss plans and when you add exercise into the equation the results can be dramatic and long lasting.

This book promises you the answers you've been looking for.

ISBN 978-1-950921-11-9
90000
9 781950 921119

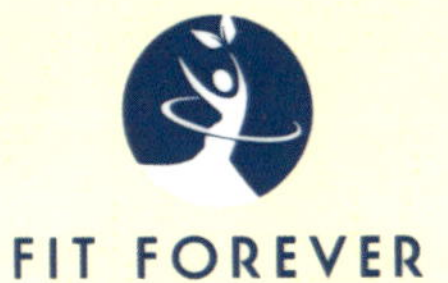

FIT FOREVER

SOMATIC THERAPY FOR SENIORS

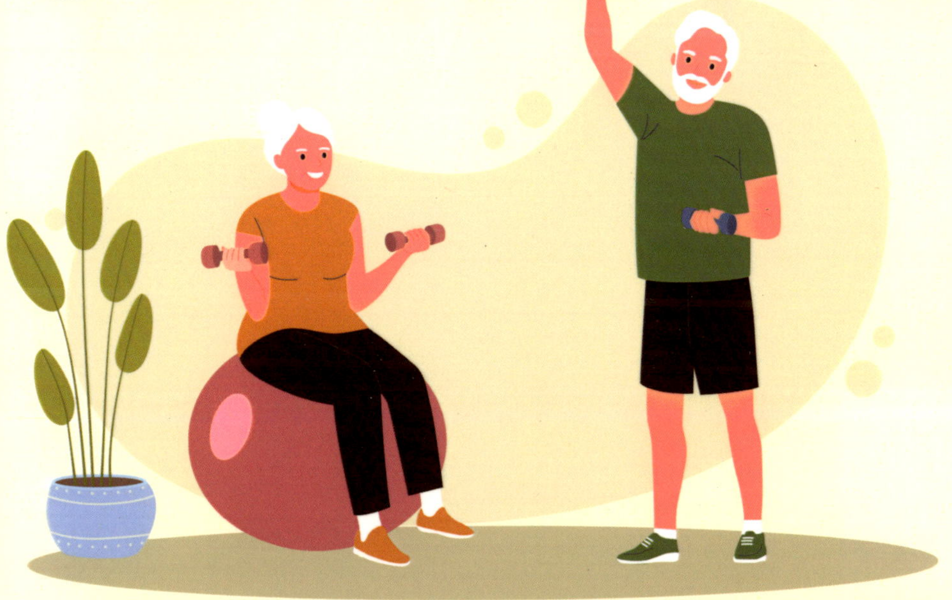